# A HUNDRED YEARS OF DECEPTION

# A HUNDRED YEARS OF DECEPTION

## WHY GARDENING MUST CHANGE

RANDY RITCHIE

Copyright © 2023 Randy Ritchie

All rights reserved.
No part of this book may be reproduced or used in any manner without the prior written permission of the copyright owner, except for the use of brief quotations in a book review.

All images by Randy Ritchie

Paperback: ISBN 979-8-9887625-0-8
Ebook: ISBN 979-8-9887625-1-5

NEXT GENERATION PUBLISHING

# Dedication

*To* Emma, Natalie and Sarah,
I am blessed and grateful to be one of your parents.
I hope this book helps shine a light on how the world might change for the better and offers a brighter future to your generation and beyond.
I love you all…

*As I held Alan's compost in my hand,
I could feel the life moving and breathing
inside my closed fist.
I knew my life was about to change.*

*- Randy Ritchie*

# TABLE OF CONTENTS

**Introduction**

**Chapter 1**
TOO MUCH STUFF! ...................................................................1

**Chapter 2**
FREEDOM OF CHOICE ...............................................................7

**Chapter 3**
WASTE NOT - WANT NOT .........................................................12

**Chapter 4**
THE REAL TRUTH ABOUT SOIL ..................................................16

**Chapter 5**
THE REAL TRUTH ABOUT ORGANICS ..........................................23

**Chapter 6**
YOU'VE BEEN CHEATED ............................................................28

**Chapter 7**
GREEN WASTED ......................................................................35

**Chapter 8**
FOOD WASTED .......................................................................41

**Chapter 9**
ARE POTTING SOILS REALLY SOIL? ............................................46

**Chapter 10**
THE MOST IMPORTANT PART OF POTTING SOIL ..........................54

**Chapter 11**
THE OTHER "STUFF" IN POTTING SOIL .......................................68

**Chapter 12**
HOUSE CLEANING your GARDEN, MIND, AND SOUL ....................75

**Chapter 13**
A DINOSAUR'S LAST BREATH ....................................................80

**Chapter 14**
SMALL THINGS .......................................................................87

**Resources**

**About the Author**

# Introduction

The road for me has narrowed. It's been happening for decades as I transitioned from landscaper to eco-landscaper, then to organic farmer and composter. I founded Malibu Compost and then had to learn the ins and outs of the lawn and garden world. I saw things from the inside of the gardening and farming industry that shook me to my core. The Garden and AG business is set up to force people to make choices that cross the line between right and wrong. I never crossed that line in my business. It made me unpopular sometimes. I was looked at as a rebel. But I could always rest my head on the pillow at night.

A huge awakening, the biggest in my life, came for me when I almost died just over a year ago. I was rushed to the hospital as my lungs and lower extremities were filling with fluid. I didn't know it then, but I would be diagnosed with congestive heart failure from Long Covid. Apparently one night, during Covid, I had coughed so badly that I'd had a heart attack.

I remember looking at my wife's face as they wheeled me through the double doors on the way to the elevators for the Cardiac ICU Unit. I was overcome by a sadness and the striking reality that this may be the last time I ever saw the love of my life. I went into prayer and meditation and never stopped. At one point everything got very still. I could hear only my labored breath and the sound of all of the medical equipment beeping and taking analysis. Then suddenly a deep, calm, intuitive thought blotted out everything... "Tell your truth." I knew it was a message from God, but I had no idea what it meant.

In the morning, the orange glow of the sun peeked up from behind the Santa Monica Mountains. I'd made it... I was going to live! An overwhelming feeling of gratitude filled me. For the next two days they kept removing more and more fluid from my body. On the third day an intense, beautiful Middle Eastern man burst into the room, "Listen Young Man, you are most likely going to die if you don't listen to me. Do you understand? Why don't any of you guys listen to me? The ones that do live. The rest of you die. Am I making myself clear? I don't need any new patients! I'm interviewing you. Do you understand? I've looked at your heart. I've read your chart and gone over everything. If you want to live you'll listen to me. Do you understand?"

Wow! He hadn't even taken a breath throughout his whole speech. "Yes Doc, I want to live. I will do exactly what you say." A wry little smile came over Dr's A's face. "Good then. We're going to try this out. I'm agreeing to be your cardiologist and you are agreeing to be my patient. Together Young Man, you just might have a shot!" He turned as he picked up my chart and started for the door, "One last thing. I see that you are primarily a vegetarian that eats organic food and that you are an organic farmer. I also see that you have faith and believe in a Higher Power." Another almost undetectable smile came over his face as he finished his thought, "Keep doing those things because they are most likely what saved your life. The organic food, working on your farm, your beliefs plus the treatments that I am going to give you are going to give you the shot at a long life."

Without another word Dr. A walked out the door. That was my first inkling of what God had given me in my prayer.

The final answer came on a flight back from a trade show three months later. I had an almost out-of-body experience as I looked at all of the poisons and toxins and fake organic products that were being sold in the big convention hall by corporations from all over the world. I had seen it all before, but this show was different for me. I saw the open and unashamed peddling of poison much akin to the drug dealing on the streets of Portland and San Francisco. It all felt so wrong to see the blatant disregard for life and the sheer brazenness of the global Big Chem companies pushing their false narrative — that somehow, some way they were making your garden better! Nothing could be further from the truth.

I couldn't stop thinking about all of the poisons, the lies, the greed, and the damage that had been done to gardens, the ecology and farms for decades. The sleeping passengers on the plane were the perfect metaphor for how gardeners and farmers had been lulled to sleep for a hundred years. Suddenly, an outline started pouring out of me. The thoughts coming faster than I could type them down. I was being given a download and my fingers struggled to keep up with the dictation.

On that flight home I was given two books to write and a new educational and consulting model to teach people the truth about gardening, health, real organics, food, farming and to use my God-given skill as a writer, to tell my truth. I had been given the truth that God wanted me to share and now I am sharing it with you.

Here is book number one…

# Chapter 1

## TOO MUCH STUFF!

On New Year's Eve of 2010, the Dow closed at 11,578. Investors in the Stock Market couldn't wait to ring in the new year. The market had gained 11% since the close in 2009. Last year the Dow hit an all time high of 36,799 on January 4, 2022.

    I know this is an odd way to start the first chapter of a "gardening" book, but as somebody who follows the market and financial news so that I can better predict and project things as the CEO of a soil company, it is the best example of how we, the world, has gotten too big and the citizenry of the western world has too much stuff. To finish my thought on the Stock Market, over the ten year period from 2012 to 2021, the annualized rate of return has been 14.8%. That's a big number. The fifty year mark from 1972 to 2021 is 9.4%. In that time the Dow went from 10,000 to 36,000. So, as you can see since the end of our last recession, The Great Recession as it was called, the financial markets have shot upwards, individual wealth has skyrocketed and the accumulation of things through consumerism has been at an all time high.

So, what does this have to do with gardening? Everything! More tools. Soils. Fertilizers. Gardening books. Plant hybrids. Garden shows. The lawn and garden industry has fed right into the global slush fund of the western world, and as gardeners, many of us have joined this rank and file spend, spend, spend, more, more, more.

I am guilty of this. How many organic coffees do I need on the coffee shelf? I counted twelve this morning. Do I really need twelve organic coffees? I can say the same thing about the stuff that my wife and I found in our old garden shed as we prepared to move to Oregon from California last year.

We had two and three of the same item buried beneath the other stuff that we had stuffed into an 6'x10' Tuff Shed. Four watering cans. Nine shovels. Many of them were different sizes and shapes and had different functions, but three were the exact same shovel and model. That company should have sent us a Christmas card!

We found stacks of speed trays, old pots from houseplants that have been upsized and repotted from our previous move, bird netting still in the package, three different kinds of knee pads. I know that my knees aren't what they used to be, but two of those knee pads I hadn't used in years and one was covered in dried Tanglefoot! You see my point, I have been a part of the buy-like-there's-no-tomorrow syndrome that has swept the garden economy.

So, why do we have so much stuff? Why do we need so much stuff? The answer is simple - marketing. We love to garden and the companies who sell us stuff in a very competitive market space bombard us with messaging to grab a piece of our wallets in an industry that was worth 104

Too Much Stuff!

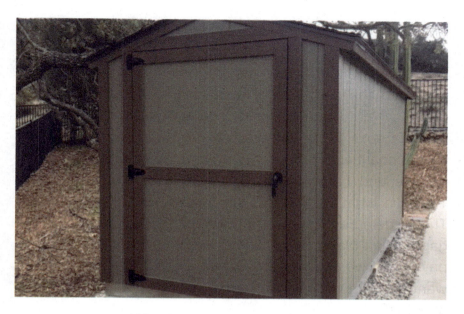

*What's in your garden shed?*

billion dollars in 2020. That is estimated to grow to 130 billion dollars by 2024. You see gardeners, we are all part of a 100 billion dollar feeding frenzy. That's billion with a "B!" That's a whole lot of rakes, shovels, bags of potting soil, seeds, plants, rubber clogs, pots, buckets, hoses, birdhouses… you name it, the list goes on.

And with all of those products comes manufacturing, packaging, labeling, shipping, merchandising and oh yes - marketing. We all get the pop-up Ads on Facebook and Instagram. The boards on Pinterest. And now, the quick videos on TikTok. It's 24 hours of gardening on demand at Youtube, Netflix and the cable channels. The manufacturers support this content with Ad Money for Ad Buys. We buy everything we can, like the good consumers we've all been trained to be, and plan for our next buy while we're still at the cash register or the online checkout paying for the current buy.

We were in this cycle until the Pandemic came along and disrupted the purchase of many of our favorite products. Supply chain disruptions due to lack of drivers, lack of fuel, lack of trucks, plus freighters for as far as the eye could see off the coast with nowhere to offload. The nurseries, garden centers and hardware store garden shops had to adapt. They did what they had to do to deal with the Pandemic. They ordered anything and everything they could to fill in the gap. I don't blame them. They have mouths to feed, bills to pay. And if we, the garden consumers, couldn't get what we wanted from them, we were taking our credit cards elsewhere.

But something happened during the social distancing and pickup lines for call-in orders to the nursery. The economy couldn't hold the weight it had gained on a diet of stimulus checks and government spending sprees. We learned that shutting down an economy isn't as easy as flipping a switch, and that somewhere along the line, we lost millions of workers. Fuel prices and transportation costs became too costly for all of the garden nic-nacs to be shipped all over kingdom come at a reasonable cost. Things like tools, soils, liquid fertilizers and pesticides suddenly became too heavy and too costly to ship. During the Pandemic the distributors were getting monthly, sometimes weekly price increases from their manufacturers and trucking companies. They had to pass those on to the stores. Those price increases haven't come down and I don't believe that they ever will even though the Pandemic is over.

Economic forecasts show in some of their forecasts slight fluctuations down on the trucking, fuel and labor that it takes to ship heavy items, but the long range outcome is that those prices are never coming back down to pre-pandemic levels. It may price many of the things we've grown accustomed to gardening with right out of the market. The marketers and Ad people of the lawn and garden market are panicking, scrambling to keep your dollars coming in.

In retrospect, did we really need all this stuff to plant a tree or a tomato? Hasn't the non-stop marketing and advertising been telling us how and what we need for our gardens for too long? Years and years of it, and in all of that time has gardening really changed? Have all of the bug sprays, fertilizers and soil products really made gardening that much better? Have the plants and trees in the native areas around our cities and states stopped growing because they haven't been fed a diet of blue liquid fertilizer? The obvious answer is no.

So, why do we need all of this stuff? Well, years and years of gardening, landscaping and farming have taught me that we don't. That idea flashed across my mind over the past several years, that just like the paradigm shift that happened to me as I switched from landscaper to farmer, I had been doing it all wrong with poisons, chemicals, bad soils and equally bad methodology and protocols. Maybe it was the same for gardening. In the blink of an eye, I realized that we've all been doing it all wrong since the NPK chemical fertilization take-over of gardening after WWI and WWII. Maybe it was time for us to take our yards and plots back, and garden the way nature intended, and not the way some gardening sub corp or shell for a chemical company has been telling us to.

# Chapter 2

# **FREEDOM OF CHOICE**

Agriculture and gardening are joined at the hip. They always have been and always will be. In 1913, the world of agriculture changed forever. Well, hopefully not forever, and hopefully this book will change not only gardening, but agriculture, back to its natural state, the place that was given to us in God's creation.

I believe that most gardeners, like most people, are inherently good. That means that they are wired to do the right things for themselves and others. For gardeners, this means that they believe what they are doing as gardeners is noble, a good thing for themselves, for others and for the planet. I also believe that if gardeners knew the history of modern fertilization, and the damage a century of chemical gardening has done to the Earth, that they would gladly put down their fertilizers and learn better ways to grow their gardens.

In 1913 Fritz Haber and Carl Bosch invented the Haber-Bosch process. Their process transformed nitrogen in the air into fertilizer. As most gardeners know, plants need nitrogen, potassium, phosphorus, water and sun to grow. In nature plants die, branches break, leaves drop, animals poop and as all of these things decompose, these three major nutrients are drawn up by the plants as they need them.

What Haber, a chemist, and Bosch, an engineer figured out was that under enough pressure using natural gas as a source of hydrogen, they could separate the bonds between the atmospheric nitrogen atoms in the air and force them to form ammonia. Ammonia became the building block for not only modern fertilizer, but also explosives and bombs which helped Germany become a super-power during WWI. One of the scariest things to me about this whole development in food production was that these two German scientists were coerced by a big contract that was dangled in front of them by BASF, a huge german chemical company.

BASF, or Badische Anilinund Sodafabrik which translated means - Baden Anline and Soda Factory, started in 1865 in Manheim, Germany to set up gasworks and street lighting. I guess "gaslighting" is an appropriate term when you consider the damage they've done to the ecology, to the human body and to the soul and soil of this planet. A quick look at the BASF roster of products finds MDI (diphenyl methane disccyanafe), Caprolactam, Adipic Acid Polyamide 6+6.6, Ammonia, Nitric Acid, several Sulfur & Chlorine products, Inorganic Salts and Urea. Many of these chemical-based products have been used to create fertilizers or are key ingredients in fertilizers, many that are still in use today.

BASF is a publicly traded corporation. Over 70% of its shares are held by institutional investors. In fact, the biggest institutional firm, BlackRock, owns over 5%. If you don't know who they are, it's worth your time to look them up and research them a little. They "manage" over $10 trillion dollars in their portfolio. There is currently a little over $100 trillion dollars in circulation around the world. That means that BlackRock "manages" a tenth of the world's money. BlackRock is a large shareholder of Apple, Microsoft, Amazon, Google, Tesla, United Health, Johnson and Johnson, Coca-Cola and Goldman Sachs.

In the lawn and garden sector, they own shares of Scotts Miracle Gro, Bayer and Conagra. I think it is also interesting to note that BlackRock is the third largest shareholder of Waste Management, the global leader in green waste. It's biggest shareholder at 9% is The Vanguard Group with The Bill and Melinda Gates Foundation second at 8.69%. BlackRock owns 7.5%. These are interesting little tidbits, right? Not so little... The Vanguard Group is one of the three Index Fund managers who control corporate America. The other two of the Big 3 are BlackRock and State Street. Ironically, or not, the biggest shareholders of BlackRock are The Vanguard Group and State Street! They are custodians of the BlackRock stakes for their investors.

The final thought on BASF is one that pertains to my "joined-at-the-hip" comment that started this chapter. BASF now owns the former Bayer Crop Science technology. Bayer Crop Science is famous for the Liberty-Link® Herbicide-Tolerant System. Liberty-Link® Soybeans create high yields and "crop safety" as their description states on their website, through "built-in" tolerance to their "fast-acting" herbicide that kills 120 weeds, grasses and glyphosate-resistant weeds. Some of their other line of science-fictionesque crop products are InVigor Canola®, Credenz Soybeans® and ILEVO® seed treatment. None of these things are good. All of these things and the money trail of billions of dollars lead us back to our german scientists.

Not only is the Haber-Bosch method responsible for all kinds of environmental damage to our air and water, which is where most chemical and synthetic fertilizer ends up, Haber and Bosch are also part of another sinister run. Our boy Fritz Haber is known as the father of chemical warfare. He weaponized the use of chlorine and other gases during WWI.

So, back to my original point in this chapter... if a gardener knew the facts, would they still want to use fertilizers, pesticides and herbicides in their garden? Not to mention the toxins that show up in conventional soils and "natural" fertilizers? When you have a globe fertilized by poison you have a globe that needs to be restored. It's obvious to me that big chemical companies don't have any of our best interests at heart when it comes to the stewardship of the Earth, especially our little garden plots or beds of roses. They don't care if your apples or plums are filled with poison. They just want you to buy more fertilizer, pesticide and herbicide to keep the profits high and their board of directors happy.

Think about it for a minute. I have for a lot of minutes. You, John or Jane Gardener go to the nursery and load your trunk up with six bags of potting soil or planting mix, two bags of compost, a bag of mulch and some fertilizer. You think you're doing something good, something noble, something that is going to help grow your plants, maybe sustain your family with food and beautify the planet. What you don't know is that if the bags of your favorite soil have conventional Ag by-products in them from chickens or green waste from global municipal waste companies, then you are putting toxins and chemical residues into your soil from the old Haber-Bosch system of growing. This will uptake into the green leafy tissue of your plants, which is horrible for a food garden. Even worse, will kill off biology in your soil, and will filter chemicals down into the aquifer where water collects, moves and ultimately dissipates into the atmosphere. This water comes back to shower us and our gardens as rain and the drinking water that we need to survive.

It's a pretty scary picture isn't it? This alone is enough of a reason to never buy another chemical or synthetic fertilizer, pesticide or herbicide again, including conventional composts and "natural" fertilizers. This also means that you will probably want to stay away from their "green-washed," faux organic products as well. Those are "organic" products that are anything but organic. There will be a lot more information on that shell game later, but for now you have plenty of food for thought.

In the coming chapters, I will plead the case to rid yourself of the chemical and agricultural bondage that many gardeners are in. We all have a choice... a Freedom of Choice. This is one of my favorite thoughts, concepts and one of the best songs by Devo. Open your mind, look out at your garden and breathe. All is not lost. All can be saved. Repaired. The damage undone. That act of free will, of taking back your garden, begins with you.

# Chapter 3

# WASTE NOT - WANT NOT

In America, we throw away 140 million tons of waste annually. Of that waste, we toss out 27 million tons of plastic, 18 million tons of paper and paperboard, 14 million tons of metals, 12 million tons of wood and 8.5 million tons of yard trimmings, all destined for landfills. While some of this stuff gets recycled by municipalities, the majority, because of confusion, laziness or lack of single stream recycling, ends up at the dump. The 140 million ton number also includes other things like glass, textiles, rubber, leather, "inorganic" waste and almost 3 million tons of miscellaneous waste. However you slice it, that is a whole lot of million tons of waste.

How much of that comes from agriculture? How much from the lawn and garden industry? I would assume that a fair share of that. Let's say it's even 10%. That's 14 million tons of waste every year that goes into landfills and creates additional problems for all of us here on Earth.

The problem with landfills is that they don't go away and they aren't a long term solution to modern man's incessant consumerism. Landfills are filled with toxins which leach into the aquifer and are a significant source of greenhouse gases. Much of the waste gets broken down by organic matter at the landfill over time by bacteria, but a lot of the waste sits for decades creating all sorts of acidic chemicals. None of this is good and none of this is helping with the pollution problem that we are facing.

Landfills are also very much a NIMBY, you know, a Not In My Back Yard type of facility, like prisons, mental institutions and drug rehabs. The people that end up with landfills in their neighborhood are already being negatively impacted by pollution. For one thing, the income levels of their town doesn't afford them a single-stream recycling system. These folks also get picked on by the lack of availability of nutritious and real organic food, and the lack of quality medical care necessary to survive the onslaught of modern sickness and disease. What we have here is a nightmare for the under privileged and underserved. The bottom line is, much of the packaging - the plastics, the bottles, the boxes that bring your gardening products to you, are items that end up in landfills.

I know at my house we recycle. We are diligent to separate the recyclables, including separate containers for glass. The trash goes into a much smaller bin these days. We also do things like home compost garden waste and use worm bins to reduce vegetable and juice scraps, but that said, we are still contributing to the landfill millions of tons total and I keep thinking over and over - how do we stop this madness!

At our companies, we use poly bags that are curbside recyclable. I often wonder how many of our customers put their empty bags into the recycling bin, and further, how many even have curbside, single waste recycling in their neighborhoods? Whatever the answer, I'm sure plenty of our

1 cubic foot and 1.5 cubic foot bags have ended up at the dump. This bothers me.

As an insider in the lawn and garden market of the gardening world, I find this and the fact that we have to use plastic bags to house, transport and shelve our products a big problem. Early on we were working with our poly manufacturer who was testing compostable poly for bags. Our compost was so alive, that in the trials, the bacteria being so active, ate right through the compostable poly within days. Even though that trial was a dismal failure, our poly manufacturer continues trying to make a more durable and longer lasting compostable poly bag. Unfortunately, for now, the best bag that we have to use for the nurseries and garden centers that we sell our products to is the curbside recyclable poly bag.

The other issue that surrounds the manufacturer of our poly bags is that plastic bags, even curbside recyclable plastic bags, are a petrochemical product. They're made from oil and natural gas. Most of the poly that garden products are packaged in come from the oil and gas industry. As I discussed a moment ago, there are new bioplastics being created all of the time. The issue for many of your gardening products is that bioplastics don't hold up, and they deteriorate too quickly for any type of sustainable shelf life. This creates quite a conundrum for manufacturers like us who want to do the right thing. We are faced with the choice of shelf space and sales versus the other option; being so local, so regional, that you could only buy our compost and soil in small loose loads that would be difficult to transport. The other issue with bioplastics is that they're really expensive.

This waste issue is a huge reason that I started looking at alternate ways of delivering better products - real organic and natural products that are less expensive, with less environmental impact and more long term benefit. I am laying the groundwork for why we need to do this and will show you how as we go on this journey together. The first thing I had to do was understand that there was a huge problem in the world and in the industry I work in. Plus, I had to realize that I was part of the problem.

Further, as a home gardener, I exacerbate the problem when I order from Amazon or buy and keep buying more and more gardening stuff that creates waste that I have to dispose of. I also had to realize that I couldn't shut down an industry, I had to help change an industry. I didn't want to make gardening impossible, I wanted to help change gardening if I could. I'm a realist and I know that change, especially change for the good is hard, but that is what we must do... Change.

# Chapter 4

# THE REAL TRUTH ABOUT SOIL

As gardeners we like to eat, sleep and drink gardening. We hang out in garden chats. We're in garden groups on Facebook. We follow people who post only pictures of flowers on their pages.

We have garden hats. Garden gloves. Our favorite gardening t-shirt. A gardening dress-up shirt to wear at flower and garden shows. We join garden clubs. Read garden magazines. Watch tons of videos online about... you guessed it - GARDENING!

I'm kind of shocked that at this point in the evolution of gardening that no-one has pointed out what has become painfully obvious to me. That the gardening world is a dinosaur that is choking on its last breath of air before becoming a petroleum reserve buried beneath the surface of the place it helped destroy.

Don't get me wrong. Watching gardening shows, being in social gardening clubs and social media gardening groups is fun and all, but when you look at the information that is being shared, the questions asked and answered, the path being burned hasn't really changed much over the past 50 years. I've spoken to many gardening clubs and have been

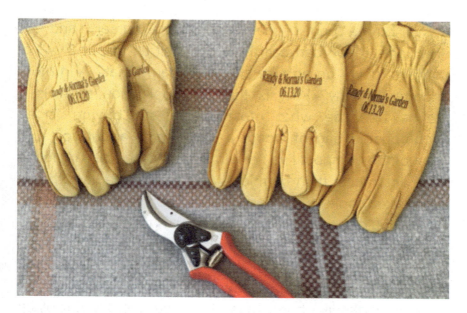

*Our monogrammed pruning gloves, one of the greatest gifts given to us by my daughter*

baffled at why the information and techniques of gardening is still mostly the same old stuff!

There are new groups of gardeners and farmers who are part of a new train of thought. They are the "fringe" of the gardening world. Unfortunately, a lot of what I've seen from the new movements of farming and gardening misses the mark when it comes to being real organic, really regenerative or sustainable. Many of the people who are in those movements have ties to conventional Ag and contributed to the issues that we have with the original organic Ag system as outlined by the NOP.

So, has anything really changed? Sadly, the answer to that question is, "No."

We buy a bag of compost at the nursery and it's directions, if you can call them that, tell us to put 3"-4" of compost down on an area of the garden. What? And more importantly, why? Why is that the application rate? Is it maybe because what most of us are buying is an uncomposted bag of wood? I don't know about you, but most of the compost I've seen in a bag or the soil yard looks more like mulch than compost. And worse, the stuff that is composted looks black, and not a deep chocolate brown like it should, because somewhere during the "composting" process it got too hot and burned.

Now, that's a radical new concept for all of you gardeners... The "burnt toast compost" theory. Your compost looks like burnt toast, because it is. It's not black gold. It's black, burnt, mostly wood with a little dirt - looking stuff that has absolutely no gold in it that I can see. By the way, you don't need to add 3"-4" of compost every spring and fall. It's overkill.

I use this example because it's one that is close to my heart. I love compost. I make really good compost, probably some of the best compost in America. To me it is like a fine wine. I love the texture. The smell. The look of it as it comes off the screen. More than anything, I love the way a great finished compost feels in my hand. If you hold a handful long enough you feel its life. I often pick up a handful of my compost, close my eyes and stand very still. Within moments, I feel the life of trillions of microscopic beings, the bacteria and fungi that are living in the compost, moving about in the living soil in my hand. It's an amazing moment where man and microbe are one. In truth we really are. The base of my compost is bacteria, just like the base of the human body is bacteria.

## The Real Truth About Soil

Did you know that there are 10 times more bacteria in our bodies than human cells? We have trillions of bacteria in us. So good, living soil is related to us much more closely than you might imagine. Maybe that's why gardeners are so drawn to the soil.

Sadly, that's not really true. I've taught thousands of people in gardening classes all over this country, and when asked, most gardeners will admit that they care more about their plants than about the soil in their gardens. In reality, all gardeners should care much more about the soil in their gardens than anything else. I know that some smarty pants out there is saying, "What about plants that don't need soil?" Okay, for you air plant gardeners - start worrying about the quality in your air. And, for you cacti and succulent gardeners - the belief that these plants don't need any compost or biology to help them grow is a garden fallacy - another one of those mis-information campaigns against cacti. I love cacti and a few cacti have actually loved me. Why? Because I gave them a little good, finished, real organic compost every year, and a nice drink of compost tea every once in a while.

The same story goes for the native plants I grow. Well they aren't actually natives, because they either came from a native plant nursery or from seed stock that I got that came from hand-sown natives, not nature sown natives. If you ask the "experts" about natives, many of them will tell you that natives want crappy soil, not too rich, just enough nutrient for barely any living creature to survive. You know what my native plants like? Well, when planting native seedlings or starts, they like about 25% of good finished compost mixed in with their native soil, and maybe a little pumice. They love that mix to start off their life in the soil

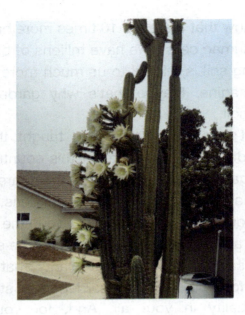
*Our large flowering cactus*

with. As they grow, they like a little showering of compost particles, good finished compost particles, tossed under them and the occasional nice cool drench of compost tea. In some larger areas of native planting, we make "snowballs" of compost mixed with water. We call them "compost bombs" and use them on our native hillsides once a year. It's really fun, I highly recommend compost bombing.

Ask any native plant you know. Give them the little bit of love that I just shared with you and they will thrive. You can always go back to the tried and true method of starving and depriving your native plants anytime you want. There you have it. I just launched another "bomb" to level years of misinformation. And the headline of the Gardening News of the World reads - "Maniac gardener says cacti, succulents and native plants love compost!"

The Real Truth About Soil

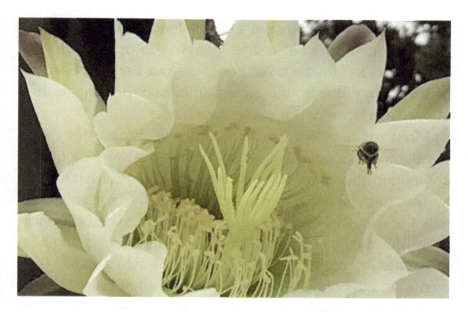

*Even the bee turned around to thank me!*

Well, that's just heresy. That goes against all of the common knowledge about cacti and natives. Well like I said you can keep on starving those poor plants. Besides that, by applying those doses of good, finished compost and compost tea to the soil around those mistreated plants, you are also feeding the biology - the microbes: bacteria, fungi and soil animals in your soil - that will multiply with a little bit of compost.

You might be asking yourself - why should I care about this? That is a good question. A fair question. The answer is simple, yet complex. It is at the root, the heart of Healthy Gardening. Feeding your soil will change the complexity of the soil and of your entire garden. When I mean feed, I don't mean 3"-4" of burnt toast put out every spring and fall. I mean small applications of good, finished, microbially- rich, real organic, living compost that will feed the life in the soil so that it can do what it was intended to do - mineralize. Those wonderful little creatures were put here on Earth to break down nutrient and mineral from decaying matter and make it available for uptake by your plants.

Most of us live on cut and fill properties from development that have killed off most of the soil biology. We compound this problem with years of chemical fertilization to feed our gardens. We need to help the soil microbes thrive and multiply. In turn, they feed more microbes which break down clay soils, add structure to sandy soils and help to naturally decompose organic matter in our gardens. They create an atmosphere below the surface that balances pH, saves water through proper dissipation and feeds our plants at the root level, the rhizosphere, with the nutrients they need to grow, thrive, ward off pests and disease, and make your garden and this planet beautiful.

Chapter 5

# THE REAL TRUTH ABOUT ORGANICS

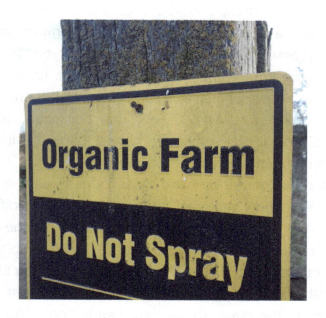

*No spray zone sign along the fence of our pasture*

I've been teaching gardening classes all over America for years now. I structured the classes around organic gardening, real organic gardening, and that meant they were centered around soil health. I realized that if I was going to upset the apple cart, I had to do it carefully and methodically. I had to start the transition to The Healthy Gardening Protocols with a foundation of teaching what real organic gardening is, and what the protocols are. That is where the story of change in the gardening world begins, understanding what real organic gardening is and how you do it?

At every garden class I teach, I always ask, "How many of you are organic gardeners?" Usually the entire class shoot up their hands! Then I ask, "How many of you eat organic food?" Usually 80-90% of the class raises their hands, with a few muttering, "I try," "As much as I can afford," "When I can find it..." I love those types of careful, under the breath commentary. It's wonderful. It's their truth. It lets me know where everybody is at. I then ask the obvious question, "Why?" This question gets a lot of participation. "It's healthier!" "Tastes better!" "It's more nutritious!" "No pesticides!"

"As organic gardeners, and as consumers who shop and eat organic... how many of you understand the difference between the $1.50/lb. conventional tomato at the market and the organic one that's $2 more?" I look around at as many faces as I can catch, "And how many of you know for sure that the organic tomato is better?" Most of the gardeners in the class shake their heads "no". "As organic gardeners and consumers who consume organic food at home, how many of you understand what it means when

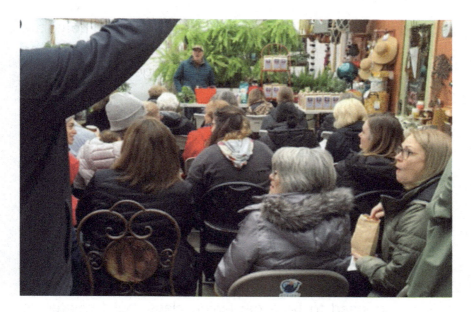
*Organic gardening class answering questions*

food, garden fertilizer, soil, soap, clothes, cotton, whatever, is labeled organic?" Not a single hand ever goes up.

Think about the information I just gleaned from asking a few basic questions from the class. I continue, "Isn't it interesting that twenty years down the road of organic certifications and hundreds of billions of dollars worth of sales of organic products and organic food, that no-one, even knowledgeable gardeners like yourselves, know what organic is?" I look around to see if they're with me. They are. I have one last question. At this point the class is really listening. Most of them don't even care that this is supposed to be a gardening class anymore. They want to know the truth. "How many of you think that because something is labeled organic it means that it is safer? And, that the government goes to great lengths to make sure that the organic products that you are buying and bringing home are better, and safer?" Someone always responds with, "I hope so," or, this vote of confidence for the huge organic money machine, "Maybe?"

My classes had no idea when they woke up that morning that I was going to shatter their organic reality. "Show of hands, how many of you really have no idea?" Everyone raises their hand in a unanimous vote that they really have no idea what the organic label means or what the actual safety and regulation of organic products really is or means at all.

I give the class some hope, "I promise you guys we will get to the actual organic gardening stuff pretty soon. I know this is supposed to be a gardening class, but I wanted to make sure that we are all on the same page, the same playing field before we get to gardening okay?" Everyone nods... we're all in agreement.

"Okay, then," I continue, "How many of you know who is in charge of labeling things organic?" More blank stares, "We've all seen the little green and white USDA Organic logo, right?" Phew. Everyone exhales as they nod "yes," we've seen that, thank goodness someone's in charge. "Anybody know what department at the USDA runs organics for the National Organic Program or the NOP of the United States?" Side to side head shaking of "No," coupled with dread that they know that they aren't going to like what I'm about to tell them comes over their faces. "It's the AMS! I'm sure we all know who the AMS is right?" More head shaking, "No's."

I smile at the class, "This is exhausting isn't it?" Everyone nods and says, "Yes." A few of my organic gardeners even laugh. "This is probably the worst gardening class ever right?" More laughter. "I think we all need a nap," I laugh myself as I finish, "AMS stands for Agricultural Marketing Services." I pause and look at everyone in the class. They all have a slightly horrified look on their faces. "Did you hear what I said, "Marketing Services...?" I hold the accent on "M," in Marketing. I can see the lights popping on behind the eyes of many in my class, so I ask the obvious, "Why marketing? Why not a specialized organic division or an organic biology department, even customer service or accounting? I mean hey why not janitorial services?" People usually laugh at that one. "Why marketing?" And then someone always utters the dreaded conclusion as to why, "Money..."

Now it is I who nod my head up and down, "That's right. Money!" I say with a hard accent on the "M." I conclude with both hands in the air, thumb and index finger rubbing side to side in the international rapper/professional millionaire athlete symbol for money grabbing, and end this portion of the class with this, "Money!"

Chapter 6

# YOU'VE BEEN CHEATED

I had no idea that when I got out of ecological landscaping and into real organic and Non-GMO composting, that I was going to teach tens of thousands of gardeners over the next decade about organic gardening, but that's what happened. I also had no idea of the realizations that I would have about organic gardening and organic agriculture being such a huge mess. Most incredibly, I had zero idea that I was going to learn many hard lessons and truths that would show me, without a doubt, that the gardening practices that we'd all been practicing and the garden industry that we'd all been following were a big fat lie. All of these experiences and realizations led me to creating The Healthy Gardening Protocols.

Did you know that organic chicken manure isn't really organic? It isn't. Unless you are raising your own chickens at home and feeding them organic food scraps and real organic laying mash, then the "organic" chicken manure that you are buying or getting in a bag is not organic. It may be labeled organic, but the places it came from and the chicken slaves that lived in squalor were on anything but an organic farm. In fact, most likely, they were in chicken hell, a jail system for animals of torture and death. The world of battery-cage chickens and fake free-range chickens, where eggs and chicken meat come from and chicken manure is sourced, is disgusting, inhumane and full of drugs, hormones, herbicide and pesticide residue, chlorine bleach, not to mention the adrenaline of fear and anxiety that these poor animals have to live with every single day of their miserable lives.

So, why isn't the chicken manure in your bagged chicken manure compost, or the composted chicken manure in your favorite potting soil or raised bed mix organic? Simple answer. Because the inputs aren't actually real organic.

What happens is companies like Somewhere Over the Rainbow Organics buy thousands of tons of chicken waste from chicken hell and then compost it, or kind of compost it. If it still stinks in your bag, it's not composted, or it's not composted correctly! Then, they add this almost compost to their soil mixes and their colorful, fun, farm-themed Hee Haw Farmhouse Compost bags and get the organic certifiers to certify them as organic. How can this be? Why would they do this you ask?

Because the NOP, the National Organic Program, allows for conventional chicken manures from conventional Ag chicken jails to be "composted." Then, because it's a natural carbon-based material, and somehow after it's allegedly "composted," it gets to be called "Organic" and for use in "Organic Agriculture" even though none of the inputs are organic. Now that folks is one amazing magic trick!

The problem grows here because of NOP Regulation (S205.203(c)(1)) which specifies that "raw" fresh aerated, anaerobic or sheet "composted" manures may only be applied on perennials or crops not for human consumption, or such uncomposted manures must be incorporated at least 4 months (120 days) before harvest of a crop for human consumption, if the crop contains the soil or soil particles (especially important for nitrate accumulators such as spinach). If the crop for human consumption does not contact the soil (eg.. sweet corn), raw manure can be incorporated up to 90 days prior to harvest. Raw solids, sewage sludge and other human waste are prohibited.

This is how conventional Ag waste gets into the organic food stream. It is also how it gets into your bags of "organic" soil, faux organic soil. Why do you think they're specifying four month and three month time frames? Is there something in that "raw manure" that could be bad, maybe dangerous?

Composted plant and animal manures (S205.203(c)(2)) are those that are produced by a process that: (i) Established an initial C:N ratio between 25:1 and 40:1 and (ii) maintained a temperature of 131 degrees F to 170 degrees F (for 3 days using an in-vessel or static aerated pile system, or (iii) a temperature between 131 degrees F and 170 degrees F for 15 days using a windrow composting system, during which period, the materials must be turned a minimum of five times. Alternatively, acceptable compost must meet the November 9, 2006 NOSB recommendations for guidance use of compost, vermicompost, processed manure and compost tea that identifies materials and practices that would be acceptable under 205.203(c)(2).

Now, it's good that we have some form of organic regulation. We don't want this to go unregulated, but what's not good, as you can see from the horses mouth, is that organic does not mean organic. Do you notice that it

You've Been Cheated

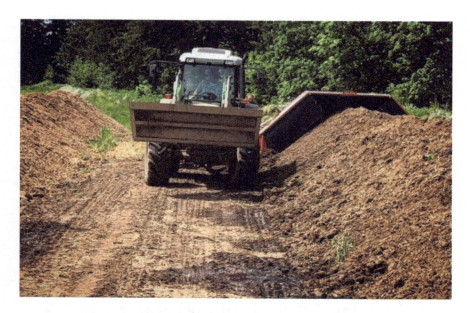

*Turning thermophilic windrows of real organic compost on a real organic farm*

doesn't say raw, composted or animal manures *from organic sources* anywhere?

I am very familiar with thermophilic composting. I've been making thermophilic and real organic compost on our farms in California and Oregon for years. The heat process eliminates pathogens, e-coli, salmonella and listeria, and the turning process aerates the compost, eliminating anaerobic bacteria which we don't want to incorporate into our gardens.

Thermophilic composting is hot composting or composting in temperatures ranging from 131 degrees to 170 degrees. I use 150 degrees F (65 degrees C) as my too hot point, and to lessen the potential for good bacterial die off. Hot composting does not break down and eliminate the chemical compounds in much of the pesticide, herbicide and fungicide residue that is in the animal waste from the feed stocks they eat. Crops like alfalfa, corn and soy are GMO crops. There are organic versions of them, but the bulk of the alfalfa, corn and soy grown now around the world is GMO. This means that they are Roundup® Ready so that farmers can spray the weeds that grow around these plants without killing the crop. The problem is that the herbicide residue is taken up into the crops. The animals eat this, poop the plant waste out and we are left with GMO-herbicide manure! And no-one, none of the soil companies test for this except for ours.

The problem gets bigger here because the NOP Regulations say that all organic products are also Non-GMO. Well that's obviously not true. If people are using conventional Ag manure or conventional plant based Ag waste that gets into the manure component of their feed or soil, then the Non-GMO claim of organic goes right out the window.

I find this horrifying. Millions of people are buying organic stuff thinking that it's Non-GMO, pesticide-free, herbicide-free and fungicide-free. They also believe it's free of all the drug residues, pharmaceutical compounds and cleaners used in conventional Ag that find their way into the organic food and organic product stream.

This is outright fraud! It's greenwashing to say something is Non-GMO and organic when it's not. The issue here is that it's greenwashing at the highest level. It's the government who is greenwashing us with standards that aren't real. The government is allowing conventional Ag a

You've Been Cheated

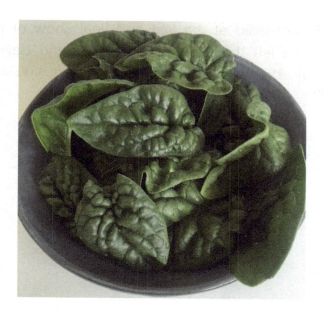

*Home grown real organic spinach never looked or tasted so good.*

seat at the organic table when there shouldn't be one to be had. Why? Why would they do that?

Because the chemical companies influence the politicians who write the laws through campaign contributions, board of director seats and speaking engagements that are worth a fortune. Greedy lawn and garden companies are allowed by these politicians to follow the bare minimum principal to distort the truth and fake you out of your hard earned cash.

Another very big influence in the gardening world is waste management. They are another big fish of deception that we are going to fry. For now, I'd like you to sit back for a minute and think about the truth that you've just been given. You've been hoodwinked. Lied to. Cheated on. As

A Hundred Years of Deception

Johnny Rotten said at the last and final show of the Sex Pistols as he left the stage of the Winterland Ballroom in January of 1978 - "Ever get the feeling you've been cheated?"

Chapter 7

## GREEN WASTED

I can't count the times over the years that I've been told by gardeners, "I use city compost! It's free!" Man oh man that sends shivers up my spine. "It's Free!" Nothing makes me crazier than the poor old church mouse mentality of some gardeners. They would rather have "cheap" or "free" than anything of quality. The soil in their garden is the proof. Nothing is free.

My grandmother, Gram as we called her, said two things that I remember. "You get what you pay for," was something she told me when she took me to Sam Ash Music looking for an acoustic guitar one summer when I was visiting her in New Jersey. I was in the throws of my big David Bowie infatuation and I wanted to learn to write songs on an acoustic guitar like him. His album, *Hunky Dory,* had a profound impact on me and still does to this day, decades after I first spun the record in my 13 year old room and now several years after his death. The world is a lot less great without David Bowie in it. The song Kooks is what I credit for making me a romantic. Google it. Give it a listen. You won't be sorry.

Back to Gram. I was taking down acoustic guitar after acoustic guitar and strumming and picking them when finally I played a D-G-A progression on a beautiful Guild D-35. It was more expensive than the Martin's and Takamine's I'd pulled down first, but it was smooth, beautiful, a work of art with a brilliantly crisp sound and deep tones. I instantly fell in love with her. I looked up at Gram. She said, "Sounds nice." I smiled, "Yeah, she's a beauty, but she's $200 more." Gram smiled back, "If there's one thing I've learned in this life Rand," she called me that endearingly, "Is that you get what you pay for." She reached out and touched my arm that was resting on the neck of the Guild and continued, "Always get the best, even if you can only afford a little, or if it takes everything you've got at the moment... get the best. You can't ever replace quality and God has a way of filling up our bank accounts and our wallets when we need more." She smiled at me with such a knowing smile that I knew she was telling my teenage self a huge truth, a secret to life. I am so grateful to have known such wise and wonderful people like my Gram and Pop. They were real. They were solid. A wave of happiness rushed over me, "Okay Gram. I'm going to buy her. It's everything I've saved up, but you're right. This is an incredible instrument... the best!"

With that we walked out of Sam Ash, me the proud owner of a beautiful Guild D-35. I learned how to write songs on that guitar and tune my voice to the music. It was an invaluable experience and purchase, one that has lasted me a lifetime.

The other thing Gram taught me was, "This too shall pass." She used to say that when times were tough, if we were suffering. She'd gotten it from her pastor who quoted

Matthew 24:35 during a sermon, and it's very appropriate for my view of real organic healthy gardening: "Heaven and Earth will pass away, but My words will not pass away." I am very much a believer. To me God's Word is the truth.

So, free city compost, let's look at that a little deeper. Besides city compost, this goes to the heart of the entire global green waste recycling and trash collecting empire. In many municipalities, the citizenry is given green bins to put their green waste into: leaf clippings, branch trimmings, dead-headed flowers, grass clippings, lots of stuff that could go into a home composting bin. This ends up in a bin which goes to the trash management company for recycling.

They put all of this yard waste into piles and start flipping it with big loaders. So far so good, right? Wrong. I forgot to mention that although a small percentage of that green waste is organic, meaning real organic green waste, most of it has petrochemical and synthetic chemical compounds or toxins and poisons all over it. That doesn't sound good does it? It isn't!

My favorite example that I share with all of my classes is the Mr. Wilson example. You know, the neighbor on Dennis the Menace? There were several episodes of him gardening. On one particular show, Dennis came over and started to bug the old, cranky retiree. "What'chya doin' Mr. Wilson?" poured out of Dennis' mouth as Mr. Wilson was spraying fungicide on his prize roses. "I'm busy Dennis fixing the mildew on my prize roses." Dennis watched as Mr. Wilson applied a thick layer of fungicide powder from his old sprayer, "Can I help?" As always, the flustered Mr. Wilson said, "No Dennis! This is very important and can be dangerous. Now please let me finish my work." Dennis leaned in over the fence and hit one of the branches, "You missed a spot right there, Mr. Wilson," trying to be helpful. Mr. Wilson lost his grip on his sprayer, it fell out of his hands, hit the ground, and as he leaned down to get it it sprayed him in the face. The camera closed in tightly on his fungicide-powder-covered face and glasses. He ended the scene by shouting out his classic line, "Martha!" calling to his wife to come out and get rid of Dennis and to help him get the poison off of his face.

Now I'm not sure if this is *exactly* how the episode went, but it's close, it's how I remember it. The point is, we all have a Mr. Wilson, or many Mr. Wilsons in our neighborhoods. And Mr. Wilson's fungicide, herbicide and pesticide-sprayed green waste ends up in the green bin, which ends up at the global green-washing waste headquarters of Trash Management Inc. It taints the entire pool of city compost that gets sold off for inputs in planting mixes and potting soils, or worse, given away as "free" compost to unsuspecting gardeners who are either too cheap or unknowledgeable to know better. Can you imagine if Mr. Wilson were around today? He'd probably be part of the class action suit against Roundup® for all of the weeds he killed with it for decades.

Here's a little tid-bit I'm happy to throw in. Scotts Miracle-Gro stock closed at $46.21 not long ago. It had hit an all time high of $244.69 on April 5th of 2021. Look at that gardeners! Why do you suppose Scotts Miracle-Gro stock has dropped over 70%? Maybe because the investors on Wall Street realized that the era of poisoning the Earth is over? Maybe the time for healthy gardening and real

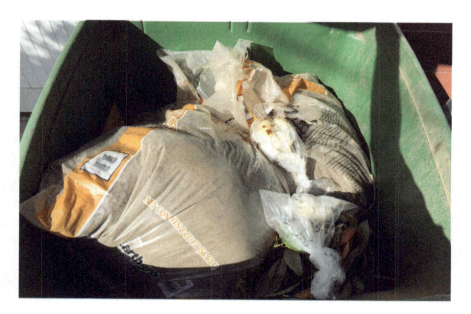

*Typical green bin contents.*

organics has come? If you think that Wall Street and the feudal lords of Big Money believe this, then you are surely into self-deception. Don't think for a second that they want real organics, healthy gardening, healthy food or a better life for any of you. They own so much of everything that they manipulate prices, company values, markets and industries at will. I checked on Scotts stock prices today and it closed at $61.40. That's up .91 today. Somebody just made a whole bunch of money and it wasn't you and me. This whole robber baron system of the Gilded Age of Tech stinks to high heaven. God knows. I know. You know.

We're going to move on to another industry owned by Big Money. The municipal food waste composting industry that is a scam and the new recycling fake out. "It's for the good of the planet," they'll tell you. What a lie. It's another way to get rid of toxic vegetable waste, cardboard and poly food wrapping with no where else to go.

One of my followers on Instagram just asked me to weigh in on their city's new mandatory food waste recycling program. She wrote asking me about what I thought of trash bins being labeled with the word "Organics," but the waste in the bin can include all food waste left-overs including KFC, fast food scraps and pizza boxes! Well, I'll throw that back out to you. What do you think?

# Chapter 8

# FOOD WASTED

The whole new zero waste idea for food waste is a really good thought, but because the premise is built on false organics, it doesn't work. If you're eating all organic fruits and veggies that either you grew at home, or you knew were grown in 100% real organic soil without GMO feed stocks in the animal's feed or pasture, and that had zero pesticides, herbicides or fungicides sprayed on them, then Bingo, Bango, Bongo... recycle it! Put it in a worm bin or food waste composting system, but without any of those caveats being satisfied, it's all a hoax - a food waste mirage of lie upon lie in the desert of petrochemical death.

The weirdest part of this whole myth to me is the lasagna layering of lies. It's like the lasagna layering or sheet mulching method of growing soil. What the heck does lasagna or sheet have to do with making soil? You don't need to layer inputs out in your yard on top of cardboard and newspaper to grow soil. You're not making a lasagna, you're making a mess. Why do it? Just put your carbon and nitrogen into a compost bin, get it moist, or use the natural moisture from your nitrogen source or rain and turn it into your static compost pile. Why do "experts," with really groovy garden hats always try to complicate things or cutesy everything up? Just compost! Please. And more importantly grow real organic gardens, lawns, orchards, trees and veggies that can actually be composted into real organic compost.

You want to layer something? You should layer your compost. Layer your browns and greens at an inch max of shredded material or broken up material at a time, not at 3"-4" where your nitrogen is going to become a wet ball of anaerobic mush. And for Pete's sake, don't use cardboard ever as part of your carbon source. Do you know if it has been sprayed with rodenticide? Or, if the glue that binds the cardboard or the wax coating is toxic?

Speaking of cardboard and as far as sheet mulch goes, in what part of biology is cardboard part of the humus equation? The answer to that question is - None! This is just another one of the many cheapo urban myths of poor man or poor woman gardening. Cardboard has binders, polymers, rat poisons, petro waste and all sorts of other garbage on it depending where you source it. Plus it takes a tremendous amount of water and nitrogen; two valuable resources we are trying to foster in the soil rather than to use to break down cardboard. Are we really too cheap to buy a decent compost or too lazy to make a decent compost at home? The cardboard might break down and disappear over time, but is that really an optimal method of disposal? Isn't that just turning our yards and gardens into landfills?

When we worked on repairing the biological balance of the Morcom Rose Garden in Oakland, CA, one of the first things we discovered was that some genius who tried to save this prestigious rose garden money, used the super-

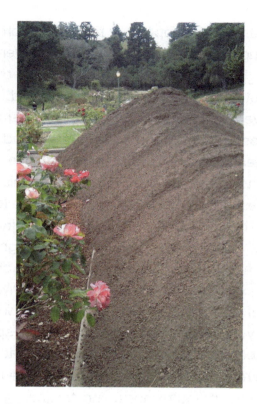

*Finished, living compost ready to be set out at the Morcom Rose Garden, Oakland, CA.*

groovy sheet mulching method of un-soil building to fix the soil on their eight acres and five thousand roses. Well, when we got there with the real organic and Non-GMO, finished, living compost that we were going to put around the base of every single rose, we had to pull up and out a 2" layer of wood mulch, which was mistake #1. Next, we found a 2"-3" layer of cardboard sheet mulch that had been there for a couple of years. That was mistake #2. It had been dumped, excuse me built up on top of the soil and was covering the crown at the base of every single rose. Can you say fungal disease waiting to happen? It had yet to break down and was choking the roses off from water, oxygen and nutrient. Great idea. We had to have our young court-ordered helpers pull it all out and send it to where it belonged... the Dump.

Once we got that garbage out of the garden, put down real compost, watered it in and did a second application of compost tea, the whole garden came alive. The bacteria, the nutrients, minerals and water turned this dying garden into the prestigious, epic rose garden of old. It was glorious. Beautiful. The microbes transformed it in ninety days back to it's glory. So here is my two cents on lasagna layering and sheet mulching - If you are doing it for weed control, stop!

In real organic gardening, we weed. "Weeds" can be beneficial if you handle them correctly. A "weed" is a wild plant that you never intended to grow in a space, and that you probably don't know of its identity. That doesn't mean it's bad. In real organic gardening, weeds are the first sign of life in the soil. If you're not going to grow anything in that spot, then the weed will build the soil for you until you do. We use weeds to add biology to the soil. We leave their roots in the ground to release nitrogen into the soil after chopping and dropping them as a cover mulch. Weeding is a great form of exercise.

Some weeds are foods with deep taproots that can access more nutrients than our average crop. For example, the leaves of the entire dandelion plant are edible and the roots can be made into a beneficial tea for you to drink.

Now let's get back to the waste that is zero waste. Non-organic, pesticide-laced food scraps, cheesy pizza boxes, anaerobic berry waste and molded cantelope brines are not exactly what you want to be composting, excuse me, food waste recycling. It's a toxic sludge cocktail that is only going to create a toxic compost that you shouldn't be growing food or anything else in, let alone be touching or breathing into your lungs.

The food waste problem is big. It is not going to get solved by a bogus recycling pick-up scheme that is run by global municipal waste management. It's a much deeper problem that starts with the toxic food chain that Big Ag and Big Food are dishing up. They are feeding us food that kills our bodies and funnels us into Big Medicine which is managed by Big Insurance who is owned and controlled by Big Money. All of this global corporate death camp runs downhill to the greed model of the institutional trading firms, billionaire corporations and the uber rich elitists who control everything.

Your independence, your freedom, your individuality, your health all breaks free when you remove yourself from the bondage of the evil entities who don't care how they control, as long as they control you. Protest by saying, "No." I will not food waste recycle or partake in your poison Ponzi scheme. If you don't start to stand up and say no, they will keep pushing you, us, the people who pay for it all until this planet is a system of AI robotica that does everything for the money masters who put them into the system to take your job, and make you obsolete. Be biological warriors who fight greed and eco-pollution starting at home, and participate in the liberation of your body, your mind and your soul.

# Chapter 9

# ARE POTTING SOILS REALLY SOIL?

Now that we know who runs the show, let's look at some of the things that Big Chem and Big Money do in the world of gardening… I'm going to break down some things that we all buy and think we have no choice. So, let's start with soil.

I'm always amazed at what gardeners accept as soil. Big bags and bales of wood, aged fir bark and aged redwood often come up as the first ingredient on a list of inputs on the back of a bag of potting soil. The list of ingredients goes from the most to the least in quantity all the way down the line. They also often begin the list with recycled forest products. That's another word for wood. Then the list goes on from the wood to include the other heavyweights in the "soil" mix: coir or sphagnum peat moss, perlite or pumice, earthworm castings, dehydrated poultry manure or composted poultry manure and sand or sandy loam. Then they go onto the fertilizers, the NPK portion of the mix: hydrolyzed feather meal, feather meal, kelp meal, bat guano, oyster shell, lime, dolomite lime, alfalfa meal and yucca. That is a lot of stuff used to create or try to mimic soil.

Let's try to break down what's going on here. The first and most obvious ingredient in 90% of all soil mixes is wood. You can see it. It's not hiding behind that pinch of crab meal in the bag. It's in your bag and first on the list of most soils because it's a cheap replacement for peat moss.

The wood, peat moss or coir constitute the bulk of potting soil mixes. This is the media component of the soil. It makes up to two thirds 2/3 of the mix. This includes about 10-15% pumice or perlite for additional aeration of the mix.

## Peat Moss

Peat moss became the universally famous soil input with Cornell University's Light-Peat Mix of 1972. Peat got a bad name back in the early 2,000's. The peat bog destruction story, like a lot of stories, is different depending on who's telling it to you. In recent years it has come under a lot of heat because of its ecological impact. A lot of folks will tell you that the peat bogs through over harvesting and mismanagement have become depleted, never to return, because they take billions of years to create. Although we're talking about peat moss here, the same can be said of soil and topsoil. I think they too, both apply to this billions of years argument. Why isn't everybody concerned about topsoil? Isn't it stripped away and washed away every day in the construction of new homes and in agriculture, never to return? Why doesn't anybody ever bring this up? The answer is because we need homes and we need food, but we don't need to strip peat bogs for potting soil and growing media. I think we need to think about both. A century of stripping topsoil through poor agricultural practices needs to stop. Feel free to bring this up as often as you'd like. I think you'll look pretty cool at a cocktail party if you say - "What are we going to do about all of the topsoil that's being depleted by Big Ag?"

The truth of the matter is that in northern Europe the peat bogs have been over harvested for agricultural purposes as well as population growth. In many northern European countries, bogs have been drained of water and the land developed and compacted for building. The bogs have been severely damaged, and are now strictly regulated.

Peat is banned in the U.K. for home gardening beginning in 2024. They are selling peat-free compost to plant in. This is interesting to me because peat is not compost and is not typically an ingredient in compost. The mixes that the RHS, the Royal Horticultural Society, give as recommendations don't look that great to me. Many of their options include coir which we will discuss later.

In the U.S. most of the peat comes from Canada. The Canadian peat industry and government strictly regulate the harvesting of Canadian peat. Twenty-five percent of the world's peatlands are in Canada; Two hundred ninety million (290,000,000) acres of peat. The entire Canadian horticultural peat industry works just fifty thousand (50,000) acres of peatland. I have a dear friend who was one of the top salesmen of peat products from Canada. His company has a very strict harvest and replant program that they adhere to. He's told me that new peat growth is 50-60% more than the amount they harvest every year.

I'm not a big peat guy, but I like to look at the facts. The fact is that peat is not the big bad wolf in the U.S. soil industry. I created a peat-based soil for our other company because of this. The soil performs beautifully. Why? Because it has 33% of a good finished organic compost in it as the humus component. Again, that's the key to any store-bought bagged or bulk soil. What is the humus or compost component of the soil?

My last bit on peat is this. I have been searching for a suitable peat alternative for years. It doesn't exist yet. You can make a pretty fair soil mix alternative with compost, wood chips and leaf mold. I use what I call the 1861 Potting Soil Mix in Healthy Gardening protocols all of the time. It's how to get away from buying bagged soils.

My big issue with most of the soil inputs, including peat moss, are the bigger picture environmental and economic impacts. That includes the question of just how sustainable is the trucking part of hauling a peat bale from Canada? I know the cost in 2022 went up 30-40%, which is a lot more than the 8-11% inflation rate. It has priced a lot of soils out of the market or to the top end of the market space. I think that so many companies are finally realizing the actual costs of hauling their cheap or free inputs just got really expensive, and that the cost of labor and fuel to process their cheap soils and faux organic soils are no longer cheap. Peat is becoming a really expensive input. That may have something to do with why it's disappearing as an input.

## Coconut Coir

The peat bog issue of the bogs being harvested and depleted caused a search for another input to be born - coconut coir. Today many soils have coir as their second ingredient, if not peat. The natural fiber, the husks of coconuts, are shredded and turned into small to large pieces that are used as media for soil. The biggest issue with coir is the salts that their exterior fibers contain. They have to be washed thoroughly, and I mean thoroughly, or buffered.

The other thing soil companies do is buffer their coir with calcium nitrate or magnesium nitrate. You cannot use buffered coir or calcium nitrate in organic farming as it is synthetic. It's made by mixing limestone with nitric acid and ammonia. Remember ammonium? Calcium nitrate is from the Haber-Bosch fertilizer mentality all the way. We see calcium nitrate used all over the landscape of farming and gardening. Both conventional farmers and gardeners use it to take care of things like blossom end rot and as fertilizer to produce larger vegetables and faster growing plants. None of this is necessary. It's toxic to animals, can harm your respiratory system, and can cause serious injury to your eyes and burn your skin. Does this sound like anything you really want to mess with?

If the coir isn't washed correctly, the EC level of your favorite potting soil could be off the charts. EC is the electrical conductivity level used to check how much salt is in a fertilizer. If the coir that your favorite soil company is buying is cheap, then it isn't washed and rinsed correctly and the salt level will hinder the plant's ability to absorb water.

Moisture is the delivery system for the fertilizers or nutrients in the soil. When you see the yellow leaves of chlorotic plants with nutrient deficiencies in a garden grown in soil with coir, this is usually the problem, a very common problem today. This isn't the only reason for chlorosis. Drainage, root issues and soil alkalinity, or soil with a high pH can also cause this.

Most of the coir in soil mixes comes over in bricks from Sri Lanka or India, which is another problem with coir. My tree hugger friends like coir for the ecological reasons of the peat bog destruction. They have happily switched to coir. I'm kind of a tree hugger myself, but I must ask my other tree huggers out there, how sustainable is shipping bales and bricks of compacted coir from Sri Lanka and India? Answer - not very! Think of the fuel, the exhaust, the spill of waste from huge cargo vessels into the sea that include garbage, synthetics, petrochemical and human waste. That's a pretty environmental picture right?

We use coir in our soil mix because of the ecological uproar over peat that became popular in the early 2,000's. We did a ton of testing and decided to go with coir because it fit the profile of our very conscientious organic customers, who are also very eco-minded and eco-friendly in their purchasing. The coir-based soil we created works really well because we wash the coir, and because our compost is a natural, real organic, Non-GMO, finished living compost that activates the simple, organic and Non-GMO fertilizers that we use. A biologically active and nutrient dense compost like ours is the main source of major and minor nutrients and trace minerals in our potting soil. The other simple fertilizers I mentioned balance that out as the plants uptake nutrient from the soil. My biggest complaint with our soil is that I don't like that coir doesn't really break down very quickly or easily. Every once in a while it can become a bit of a tangled knot in the rhizosphere of the plants. The root zone is definitely not the best place for a tangled web of Sri Lankan coir, but it does happen.

At the end of the day, I don't think that peat or coir are really sustainable.

## Perlite

Neither is the cost of mining and processing the last component used for aeration in the media portion of your potting soil. Perlite. Perlite is mined volcanic glass. In the U.S. it comes from places like Oregon and New Mexico. Large amounts of perlite are processed in China, Greece, Italy, Turkey, Mexico and the Philippines. Perlite is mined, then crushed, dried and screened. Afterwards, they ship it off to a processing plant where it cooks in furnaces at 1400-1800 degrees F (760-982 degrees C). The water gets trapped inside and the heated glass expands to the little white pieces that we see in soil mixes. Then it's trucked or shipped again and bagged. Lots of touches. Lots of trucking. Lots of costs! What historically has been a cheap input is now getting more and more expensive. How sustainable is this financially?

Perlite factories emit aluminum, calcium, chromium, florine, lead, magnesium, iron, mercury, nickel, titanium and zinc into the atmosphere. They use filters to filter the pm, or particulate matter, and Co2 emissions. They use natural gas to heat the perlite. How environmentally stable and sustainable is adding little white volcanic balls of aeration into our soil that needs to be trucked or shipped from point A to point B, C or D? The answer - not very. The picture is even worse for perlite that is shipped from other parts of the globe.

What we've been looking at here is the aeration component of the modern faux soil mixes. None of these soils, including ours, are really soils. They're a misnomer for recipes of by-products and mined and harvested items that have been thrown together to literally grow the ornamental plant industry around the world. These soils are nothing more than a Rachel Ray cooking show, no, a Julia Childs episode of The French Chef, her classic 60's cooking show. Can't you hear Julia doing a gardening class on tv, "Now we drop the peat into the bucket of fir fines and stir slowly to mix the entire batch... evenly and smoothly." She then reaches down and picks up a bowl of perlite and shows it to the camera, "Now we add the finishing touch, the creme de la creme, the tour de force of the aeration of potting soil, mined or crushed perlite, oh and if you haven't any, you can add a little rock. Pumice will do nicely." She drops the perlite gingerly into the mix and, "Spread it lightly, evenly, then whisk it into your batter of wood and peat to create the base of a beautiful New York Cornellesque potting soil mix!" As she whisks it in, the camera pulls back to reveal a garden-gloved Julia happily whisking away, "Oh I love how fluffy and light a good, delicious potting soil can be... it's just scrumptious!"

That's not exactly how the guys at the soil yard mix your favorite potting soil, but the intention is accurate. The bottom line is that it's not soil! None of the ten's of millions of bags of this stuff sold every year. It's a cake recipe. It's a waste batter of stuff that creates stuff so that you can plant a plant into a hole and force it to grow with fertilizer.

In this chapter, we've just covered 2/3 of your soil recipe. Next we're going to get into detail about the humus component of soil recipes. I just heard Julia in the back of my mind, her wonderfully shrill voice calling out, "Did you just say soil recipe? I love it!"

Chapter 10

# THE MOST IMPORTANT PART OF POTTING SOIL

The most important input for all of the artificial and faux potting soils is the one that they never get right - humus. The humus component of homemade soils and store bought potting soils and planting mixes comes from the compost that is added to the recipe. No more Julia Childs jokes! This is serious business with me because this is where most soil recipes fail. This is where the amateur soil chefs, the cheap corporate soil makers and the creepy faux organic soil slingers will never beat Bobby Flay!

What we use in soil mixes to create the humus component is compost. Humus is the latin word for earth or ground. Humus is created by the decomposition of plant and animal material in nature. It is organic soil matter in nature in the truest sense. This means that there are no inputs other than leaves, twigs, decaying stems and branches, dead grasses and animal feces and urine from critters scurrying across and flying above the Earth. Humus has the major and minor nutrients in it and is full of minerals. It also retains moisture which helps seeds to germinate, plants to grow and aids in the delivery of nutrient to the root zone of plants for uptake.

This is why the forests, wetlands, grasslands and woods in nature don't need a fire fighting air tanker to fly over them in secret at night, to drop chemical salt-based fertilizers that look like a 1980's aqua blue cocktail from the Tom Cruise movie "Cocktail" to survive. They survive through the process of mineralization, which is when soil microbes - bacteria, fungi, algae, protozoa, nematodes, earthworms and soil animals like spring tails break down the nutrients and minerals in the decaying and decomposing organic matter in soil into a form that they can uptake.

These soil microbes and microorganisms are the single most important link to humans and healthy food via healthy soil. If there is one thing that every gardener should be prioritizing, it's not growing a prize rose, or the biggest tomato in the neighborhood, not that there is anything wrong with growing a big tomato or a prize rose, but fostering, growing and caring for the biology, the microbes in your soil should be job one, priority number one for every gardener. These microorganisms do so much besides feed plants. They help regulate and adjust the soil pH, protect plants from disease, preserve the ecology by consuming greenhouse gasses like carbon dioxide, methane and nitrous oxide, and purify water by removing pollutants. There are more soil microbes on this planet than people. In fact, there are more microbes in a teaspoon of living soil than humans on Earth.

Now, let's get back to your favorite potting soil or planting mix and let's look further at the humus component; that portion of the mix at a minimum of any decent soil should be twenty-five percent, but in reality more like one third. Most of the faux organic soils have dehydrated poultry manure, composted poultry manure, green manure, green waste compost, earthworm castings or sand as their humus component of their soil. By the way, sand is not a humus component. It's a super cheap filler. Washed sand has no nutrient value at all. The only value I can see as to why some soil manufacturer puts sand in their potting soil mix is for drainage... and that's a stretch folks.

## Steer Manure Compost

Steer manure is absolutely the worse thing you can put anywhere in the garden. I shudder every time I pass by a depot and see gardeners putting bag after bag of this in the back of their pick up trucks or in their trunks. It seems to me like they can never get enough steer manure. The same goes for the weekend warriors who buy their half pallet to a pallet and throw it in their buddy's pick up so they can stink up the neighborhood. That, along with some bottles or bags of chemical fertilizer so that they have the greenest lawn in the state! Who cares about having the greenest lawn in the state? I would be impressed if they wanted to have the healthiest lawn in the state.

Steer manure comes from the worst of the CAFO operations. Those cows on their way to the slaughterhouse know what's coming. They can smell it. I've been there and I've seen the fear in their eyes. Why would you want to put something in your yard that came from a killing mill? Is that the kind of energy that you want to be putting into your garden? Don't ever buy a bag of steer manure ever again. The only way that we're ever going to change the way we treat animals on this planet is to quit buying their by-products. When we do that we tell Big Ag we're not co-signing the way you treat animals anymore.

So you know, steer manure is full of salt, high in ammonia and is loaded with toxic residue from herbicide that come from the GMO feed stocks; the alfalfa and soy that they are fed. If you want to do something heroic, go to your local depot or nursery and tell them to quit selling steer manure because you don't like how the animals are being treated.

Steer manure is not the same as dairy cow manure and dairy cow manure is not the same as organic dairy cow manure. Organic dairy cows must graze on pasture for a minimum of 120 days per year, per grazing season. Conventional animals never see a pasture and are fed GMO corn, soy and alfalfa. Don't use any manure ever that isn't 100% organic.

## Chicken Manure Compost

So let's have a look at the other compost or humus components I listed that we find in most conventional soil recipes and in many of the faux organic ones. One of the biggies is dehydrated chicken manure or "poultry" manure as proper folks call it. My favorite misuse of terminology when it comes to chicken manure is - aerobically composted poultry litter.

The first thing to do with any animal base component of soil is ask yourself, "Where did it come from?" If the chickens were raised on a conventional chicken farm, then they are eating mostly corn and soy. In fact, almost half of their diet is corn and over one quarter is soy. Another big component is bakery meal. Bakery meal? Doesn't that sound yummy? Well it must be. It's one of the ingredients used to feed "poultry" which you now know is chickens on big farming concerns.

They also feed this wonderful modern food source - bakery meal - to pigs on large farming concerns. Well, this concerns me because when I heard about it I wanted to know what the heck it was! I'm sure you're asking yourself the same question. I'm glad you asked. It's a mixture of breads, crackers, chips, cookies, snack foods, tortillas, cereals, and my favorite ingredient - related food by-products. Those are all of the non-edible waste goodies from snacks mixed together, ground up and dried before it is shipped off to the big farm concerns and fed to the unsuspecting poultry who get to eat loads of this heaping helping of garbage before reaching your garden or your table for dinner.

Here's the rub with this diet. The corn and soy, as with the corn and soy in most people's diets, of Mickey D's, the Colonel and Starbucks are all from GMO crops. These GMO feed stocks are Roundup® Ready. These crops, and many others, are sprayed by farmers for weed control. The corn and soy are resistant to the Roundup®. The weeds are not, and they die. The herbicide residue stays on these crops. These broad-spectrum herbicides like Roundup® do not break down easily, which means that they are in the feed that the chickens, excuse me, the poultry eat that give you the manure for your favorite potting soil, planting mix or toxic compost. The compounds in the herbicide residue do not get "cooked out," or broken down in the "composting" process, as many who compost conventional Ag waste claim. Those compounds make their way up into the soft green leafy tissue of your veggie garden, which means you

## The Most Important Part of Potting Soil

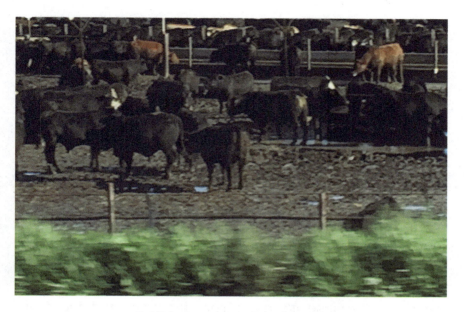

*CAFO feedlot, I-5 Interstate*

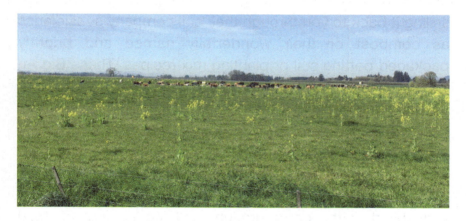

*Steer manure is not the same as dairy cow manure. Here, dairy cows roam the pasture on our organic dairy farm.*

get to eat Roundup®! Yay- now that's a wonderful closed loop system for you. That folks is why the organic registration and certification process doesn't work. You cannot allow conventional Ag waste into the production of organic foods and products, and that includes the biggest selling soil mixes, the faux organic soil mixes. They are what every single nursery in the United States sells and the big box stores blow out the door often with Buy 3, Get 1 Free specials!

Did you ever wonder how they could do that? Simple. The big soil companies get paid to take garbage and Ag waste away with what are called tipping fees. That means they get paid to haul away the toxic inputs that they are given for free. They don't pay for their toxic chicken manure because it's worthless. They get paid to haul it away from the farms because it's a problem for them that the "soil" companies solve. They take this toxic garbage back to their plants for processing, allegedly "composting," and then selling it back to you through their soil company subsidiaries as compost or their wonderfully named and brightly packaged potting soil or planting mix recipes. These Big Ag death soils are the ones that are sold everywhere and that 90% of the gardeners in America are using.

To quote Jackie Chiles, the Johnny Cochranesque attorney on Seinfeld, "This is egregious, outrageous, outlandish!" It's a complete misuse of power by the government, of marketing of the soil manufacturers and a very blind faith, corroboration and co-signing of total nonsense and fabrication by the nurseries and big boxes to sell fake organic and toxic soils to you, their customer.

## Worm Castings

Then we've got worm castings. There has been a lot of confusion over worm castings, or vermicompost, and compost in recent years. We will be using worm castings and vermicompost interchangeably throughout this book as they are basically the same thing. No-one is getting pure clean castings out there. Earthworms are grinders in nature who break up decaying roots and leaves, as well as animal feces and manures. They also eat bacteria, fungi, nematodes and protozoa, aid in the mineralization process and add to the collective decomposition and decay that creates humus.

In North America, the earthworm Eisenia fetida, common name "red wiggler," is mostly used in vermicomposting by worm farms, as well as for fish bait. This is not the deep, dark red or brown fat earthworm that you see deep in your soil, the Lumbricus terrestris. Lumbricus terrestris thrive in the soil and burrow deep into the soil, while the wigglers live in decaying organic matter and live nearer the surface of the soil in groups. All composting worms are earthworms, but not all earthworms are composting worms.

Some of you worm casting lovers will take my words as heresy, but in my years and years of working out in the field as a farmer, gardener and landscaper, I can tell you that castings are great, I love them. I use them. We have worm bins at my house, but they do not stack up in the fertilization process or soil building process to good, finished, real organic compost. There I said it. Finito.

Worm castings are another form of humus. They are a great source of nutrient for your plants, but they don't have the long-term effects that compost does when it comes to building soil structure. Castings are finer and don't have the coarseness that comes from the organic matter that compost does.

The problem with commercial worm castings is where these big companies get their inputs from. What are the worms eating? Do those companies have large, real organic farms their getting their scraps from? My family grows real organic and we use the real organic pulp from our real organic juicing to make great real organic worm castings. I know of some big worm outfits that use cardboard and shredded cardboard and garbage to feed their worms. Others feed them horse manure which comes from animals fed with GMO hay and given Ivermectin as a dewormer. The deworming agents used on horses are anti-fungal. Many horses are also given hormones and antibiotics by their veterinarians.

None of the feedstocks used by these large commercial worm operations are real organic, nor good for your garden. Create your own worm bins if you want to use castings.

## Horse Manure Compost

I grew up around horses and practiced natural horsemanship. I love horses, but I'm not a fan of using horse manure in the garden. Besides what I just wrote about them eating GMO alfalfa and being dewormed with Ivermectin, horse manure is not a very biologically processed manure. Horses eat hay and it seems like within minutes it's coming out the back end.

Their manure is hot and can be loaded with weed or invasive plant seed, because it is so porous, allowing weeds to literally blow into it. It also doesn't have the complexity of

# The Most Important Part of Potting Soil

biology or microbial diversity as my favorite manures: organic dairy cow, sheep, goat, alpaca and lama. I'll take any of those manures over horse or chicken for that matter any day.

I was at a tabling event one afternoon at a very large community garden in Los Angeles. When I say very large, I mean it. This place was huge. It was also a community garden that prided itself on sustainability and self-sufficiency. Now I've heard they're also into regenerative gardening! That's funny!

One of the crown jewels of this enormous community garden was their composting operation. The members of this esteemed community garden put it on themselves to create a giant composting operation for their giant community garden. The main ingredient of their compost was... you guessed it... horse manure.

The composting site was built into the hillside and had two giant horse poop pits where they would also add green waste from their garden plots. Apparently a local horse-boarding facility dropped off lots of manure there and the garden members would turn and water these manure pits by hand. I give them an "A" for effort on that. They had built big grates at the bottom of the pits to pull the "finished" compost out from underneath the bottom of the piles.

So, back to the tabling event. We had been invited to table and talk about compost tea and compost to its members. The tabling event was part of a community garden event for all of the community gardens of Los Angeles. There were several different tables that were talking about a variety of things including seeds, plants and drought resistance. This garden boasted several garden writers and bloggers as members of their gigantic hillside community garden. I must admit, it did have a million dollar Los Angeles view!

We were discussing the benefits of compost tea with a group of folks when out of the corner of my eye I saw an elderly gardener dragging a trash bag full of something down the trail below us. She was apparently hauling some of their prized compost down to her bed. I asked the people at our table to excuse me for a moment, then raced down the hill after the elderly gardener.

Her 33 gallon trash bag was smoldering. She had no idea and neither did any of the other gardeners who were tending their plots. I guess it was community gardening as usual. I called out to the lady, "Ma'am, Ma'am... Miss... you're bag is on fire! It's smoldering!" She finally stopped and looked down at her bag. It was now literally on fire. Smoke was billowing up off of the bag and drifting across the nearby plots.

She bent down to inspect the bag as I caught up with her. "Don't touch it. It's on fire," I said as I grabbed a shovel laying next to a plot and started smashing the bottom of the bag that was now leaking flaming horse manure "compost." Obviously, it wasn't too composted.

She yelled at me, "What are you doing?" I looked at her, "I'm putting out your compost. It's on fire." A really strange look came over her face, "That's always how it is. It's great stuff. I use it all of the time." I finally got the fire out and looked at the woman, "You use this all the time?" I asked. "Yes," she said as she started pulling the bag down the path again, "I've got to get this into my beds today. They need composting!"

Incredulous, I stood there with my mouth wide open and watched her drag the smoldering bag down to her plot. I wanted to say something, but no words would come out. I shook my head to myself with her voice playing over in my mind, "It's great stuff. I use it all the time." I sneaked a quick peak at her plot. I can tell you from the looks of it... not great stuff.

## Green Waste Compost

The last component of the humus portion of the potting soil and planting mix recipe is green waste compost. This ingredient shows up as composted green waste and composted plant material. The irony of these ingredients is that on paper, plant-based compost looks good. What could be wrong with it? Well... Here's Johnny!

How about that all of the wonderful green waste comes from the municipal recycling stream of death! Remember Mr. Wilson? As discussed earlier, pesticides, herbicides, fungicides and residue from green waste garbage get dumped, mixed and processed at the dump along with old tires, soiled diapers, dog poop, kitty liter, needles, guns, whiskey bottles and anything else that humans put into a green bin that gets carted off to the dump, I mean the municipal waste management facility.

Gardeners all across this country pour millions of tons of chemically treated leaves, grass clippings, prunings, veggie waste, flower buds from deadheading and all of the dead weeds they can round up, pun intended, into their green bins. It gets hauled off to the dump then processed, which means it's allegedly composted. The soil companies buy this green waste compost labeled "composted green waste" or "composted plant material," then add it into their brightly colored bags of potting soil and planting mix that advertise:

No Toxins, No Toxic Chicken Manure and No Animal Component. Really? How about the green soil recipe of death that you are proudly shoving into your bag? Do you think any of the "soil" companies test for pesticides, herbicides or fungicides? I guess those aren't toxins! How do these people sleep at night?

For the record, I make compost out of organic dairy cow manure, natural wood chips from the forest that are used as bedding for the organic cows on the organic dairy and the biodynamic preparations 502-507: yarrow, chamomile, stinging nettle, oak bark, dandelion and valerian. That's it. It's thermophilically made. One hundred percent finished, clean, real organic compost.

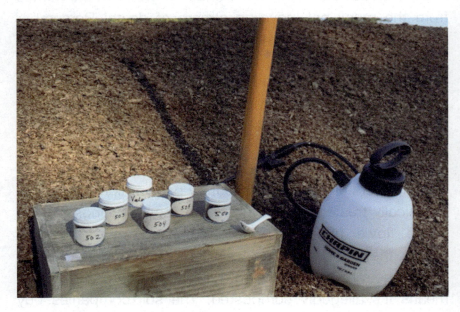

*Adding Biodynamic preparations and spraying valerian tea to real organic compost windrows*

## The Most Important Part of Potting Soil

To close on the humus component of bagged soil, bulk soil and planting mixes - the manure compost or green waste all comes as waste, as a by-product from toxic and filthy sources. Once these manures are hidden in a brightly colored bag or at a bulk soil yard in a bin with a sign that reads, "Organic Potting Mix," you have no idea that what you are buying is a toxic waste pool, not a recipe, but something that is wrong, very wrong, and that has bothered me for a long time about the lawn and garden industry. It's time to fess up people. Tell the truth. Straighten out. Get off the crack!

## Chapter 11

# THE OTHER "STUFF" IN POTTING SOIL

The last portion of your store bought potting soil or planting mix recipe is the fertilizers, wetting agents and biological inoculants... the other stuff. Stuff is a good catch-all term for all of the extras in bagged and bulk soils. Stuff from sawdust to alfalfa meal, fish bone meal, feather meal, kelp meal, endo and ecto mycorrhizae, beneficial soil microbes, dolomite lime and wetting agents are on the list of one popular brand. That list comes right after the composted green waste, the humus component that you just read about. It follows aged fir bark, fir bark, pumice and sphagnum peat moss, the media and aeration part of their soil mix.

The fertilizer part is the last part of most soil recipes. Why do we need all of this stuff? We'll get to that in a second, but first let's look at a couple more "stuff" lists, and then we'll discuss why.

Another popular brand's high-end soil has this list of stuff in it: gypsum, soft wood biochar, bat guano and worm castings. Their other popular line lists this: hydrolyzed feather meal, dehydrated chicken manure, worm castings, bat guano, kelp meal, alfalfa meal, oyster shell, and dolomite lime. On another coast they've added some new gems on their list of stuff to go along with composted poultry manure. They also add lobster and crab shell and kelp meal. The rest of their mix is mostly peat moss, almost 70% of the mix, with just a little bit of aged fir bark. Then they throw in some of the fertilizers I gave you before.

Another national brand that's popular these days has limestone, earthworm castings, alfalfa meal, kelp meal, feather meal and yucca extract. It also has endo and ecto mycorrhizae in it. They market it as enhanced with Myco-Fabuloso! It's not actually called that, but it's close enough. So the multi-million dollar question is, "Why?" Why do the soil companies have to put all of this stuff into their mixes? The short answer is... they don't. If they had a good, finished, real organic compost, then they wouldn't need all of this stuff added into their mix. Many, no, almost all of the potting soils on the market are made from Big Ag's conventional animal by-products and Big Trash's waste recycling bin garbage. Is garbage what any of us really want to be growing anything in? Is garbage really something that we want to pay for and bring home?

Aren't we just turning our gardens into garbage dumps when we do that?

I am telling you this, because I have grown tired of all the closed loop garbage dumping, faux organics and Big Ag lies that make it to our gardens and onto our tables. One of the purposes of this book is to tell the truth about the toxic garbage and waste that makes it into the food you eat and into your plants via toxic products: fertilizers, compost and soils. I am all for recycling and composting. What I'm not all for is the lying and deception that the lawn and garden industry dances around by literally taking trash from Big Ag and Big Waste and then talking it up with all sorts of flowery, phony marketing and advertising campaigns, then dumping this junk into pretty poly bags and packages to trick you into buying it. This leads you into a false sense of security that you're getting real, clean, safe, healthy, honest-to-God organic and ecologically sound products, when you're not! It's a crime.

The whole system is based on falsehood after falsehood and nobody is saying or doing anything about it. Well, I am, because I can no longer stomach the stealing of your money by a totally phony and bogus green industry. The only green I see in much of the lawn and garden industry is billions of your hard earned green spent on bags, boxes and bottles of chicanery.

If a robber comes into your house and steals your stuff, you want the police to catch them, get your stuff back and lock them up, right? In this case the robber, the industry, is literally stealing your money, and the police, the government, is in on it, so much so, that you, John or Jane Gardener don't even know you've been robbed. Well now you do. I've spent thirty years in this industry and I am writing this book to tell you that you're being robbed. Now, that's the bad news. The good news is that I have a solution for you and it's called... Healthy Gardening. In my other book, I teach you how to use real organic minimal inputs and the Healthy Gardening Protocols.

Let's wrap up the detective work with a look at all the "stuff" that's in your potting soil; the meals, the powders and the inoculants that you absolutely 100% don't need. To do this, we'll go back to the scene of the crime, the list of ingredients on the back of the bag.

## Feather Meal

Let's start with feather meal. It shows up as hydrolyzed feather meal, or just good old feather meal. Remember what those poor birds are eating, the main portion of their diet is GMO corn, soy and snack foods from that fabulous bakery meal? It's all GMO, Roundup® sprayed goodness. That makes any chicken by-product manure in a bag a big NO, a nada, a not in my garden component - ever!

## Bone Meal and Blood Meal

That also goes for bone meal and blood meal. Same thing. Why do we need these CAFO (Concentrated Animal Feeding Operations) inputs in our gardens? First of all CAFO's are basically jails and prisons, no they are concentration camps for Big Ag meat, dairy and eggs. They house those poor animals in terrible conditions, feed them a diet of poison and then kill them - with little care for the fact that they are living beings that God created. They do this just because they are a part of the "food chain." Big Ag treats them as things and not beings. It's time to awaken to where your food comes from, and secondly where the animal component of the fertilizer for your gardens comes from. Stop co-signing the brutality and horrid stewardship of this industry. I hope that by now you're starting to see the barbarism and criminality of all of these interrelated and joined-at-the-hip industries, and that you never want to give them another dime. As Morrissey once wrote, *Barbarism*

*Begins at Home.* Do you really want any part of their brutality?

Do your plants really need a 3-15-0 or 4-12-0 bone meal from scared, tortured animals to grow? Or a 12-0-0 blood meal from death factories to grab their nitrogen from? No! No! No! It's an absolute lie.

## Alfalfa Meal, Soy Meal and Cottonseed Meal

While we're still on Big Ag, let's look at what else you don't need from them: alfalfa meal, soy meal and cottonseed meal. These are all GMO crops, even worse, with alfalfa, they can use the herbicide at any time for weed control but also to get a taller stiffer stand for cutting and for more tonnage at harvest. That means horses, cows, goats, sheep, any animal eating conventional alfalfa is getting an extra helping of herbicide. Guess where that herbicide ends up?.. In your garden!

Soy is another big GMO crop. Don't use it. There are a couple of exceptions with alfalfa and soy meals that are organic and Non-GMO. We have used these, however be careful because 99% of what is on the shelf is conventional and genetically modified.

As far as cottonseed meal goes, cotton is one of the most pesticide-heavy crops grown in the world. Cotton is the filthiest crop on the planet in terms of pesticides. 2.5% of the cultivated land on this planet is cotton and 16% of the pesticides used on the Earth each year are for cotton fields. The pesticides used in cotton production have been found in ground water all around the world and are poisonous to both humans and animals. Enough said. Do you want to bring cottonseed meal with toxic residue on it into your garden? You've been warned.

## Fish Meal, Fish Bone Meal, Crab Meal and Shrimp Meal

The last of the stuff are things like fish meal, fish bone meal, crab meal and shrimp meal. The question here is where did the fish or crab or shrimp come from? Are they wild caught or farm raised? The fish kibble that farm raised fish eat are called pellets. They come from fish meal, fish oil and plant and animal trimmings. That doesn't sound very natural does it?

Farm raised fish are kept in unnaturally dense concentrations within tanks, and pollutants and nitrates can build up in water. It closely resembles factory farming of terrestrial animals. In order to induce breeding, farmed fish are injected with hormones. There are a number of terrible things that the fish are put through after that, which resembles a horror film or nightmare. Buy wild caught only.

One last thing on fish. East Coast v. West Coast. I prefer cold water, East Coast wild caught sourced if I need some. The same goes for kelp meal or liquid kelp.

## Mycorrhizae

Stuff like endo and ecto mycorrhizae is fine, but is it still alive in the bag when you get it? And in reality did they really add that much at all in the first place? Most companies are using this as a greenwashing tool to steal your green, and when they make up cutesy names like Myco-Fabuloso, C'mon now people, you weren't born yesterday! Why do you need to buy the potting soil that advertises Myco-Fabuloso on it? You don't!

I add mycorrhizae in the soil or beds when planting, not in potting soil. Get it from reputable companies.

## Dolomite Lime

Soil companies add lime to potting soils and mixes to raise the soil pH. Why do so many potting soils need to have their pH raised? The answer is because the ingredients in them make them too acidic. In nature, pH is adjusted by microbes. This tells me that most of the soils in the pretty multicolored bags don't have much biology in them, don't have good, finished, real organic compost in their stuff and are wood and peat-heavy. They need a large humus component like compost to stabilize their pH. Rather than adding dolomite lime to their mix, they should add a good, finished, real organic compost. The microbes will take care of the rest.

## Wetting Agents

The last piece here is wetting agents. Does soil in nature need a wetting agent? C'mon now!

The main thing with all of this stuff is that it's fluff & fold garbage to make you think you need it in the potting soil to make your plants grow. I have fallen prey to this misconception myself, but those days are over.

# Chapter 12

# HOUSE CLEANING YOUR GARDEN, MIND, AND SOUL

Now that you know what's in all of the products you've been buying and using, it's time to talk about the people who've influenced you to do so. I want to discuss the "experts" and influencers of the gardening world. This should open up a whole set of new doors of perception for all of you gardeners as we start to clean house.

Think about how gardening would look like to you without fertilizers, pesticides and fungicides. I want you to consider how much money you've spent on sprays, dusts, powders, pellets and crystals to get rid of bugs or disease, or to N-P-K your garden over the years. It's probably a lot of dinero, that's money in español.

I wanted to open up the gardening world of gardeners to everything we don't need in the garden or to garden with. I figured that would be a great way to start a housecleaning, well a garden shed or garage cleaning of everything that we have been taught or told we need from gardening influencers who love their turf builder or planting in my favorite oxymoron - Scotts Miracle-Gro Organic. We've also learned gardening tips at garden shows, garden clubs, social media ads and master gardener programs, as well as from PhD's and the hat people... the garden "experts." Did you ever stop to consider what makes the hat people "experts"? First, they have their brand, which is their hat, and their hat says, "I garden, therefore I'm an expert." It's kind of a weird play on Rene Descartes' principle published in 1637 of his translation of the latin phrase Ergo Sum, "I think therefore I am." Most of the "experts" are just slinging around recycled garden notions for money. They get sponsored by the big chemical or faux organic companies to recycle the gardening myths and legends that built the modern gardening industry. They make sure that the money keeps flowing in.

If you don't believe me, go on any of their websites and read their blogs. See how many products they list in the blog or how many ads pop up alongside the text or on their header. Look for their sponsors or the words, "Sponsored by." Garden "experts" are stooges for the purveyors of poison and false knowledge, wrapped up in a homey, landscapey, gardeny outfit with a hat. Still don't believe me? A stooge is a noun defined as: A person who serves merely to support or assist others, particularly in doing unpleasant work. I'd say that hawking poison and false ideology is definitely unpleasant work. I hope this doesn't seem too harsh, but I've been giving you the very unpleasant truth of the companies and corporations and now influencers of our favorite pass time. I'm sorry but to me anyone who purports to be an "expert," but doesn't have a deep understanding and awareness of where much of the information came from that they are teaching, lecturing and posturing about is not much of an expert. You've got to know if you're an "expert' that Big Money, funneled through Big Education to study, test and approve the chemicals that Big Chem wants to use, influenced your thoughts and concepts. If you are going to teach and lead people in the world of gardening, you better know this. I think that's a good jumping off point for your housecleaning.

The first thing that you don't need in your garden is 95-100% of the garden garbage that any stooge has recommended. The caveat here is this, if someone recommends something for your garden that is actually microbial or biological in nature, is not from a sub corporation or company owned by a huge chemical outfit, waste management entity, or a faux organic operation who gaslights the public with greenwashing, then it would be a good idea to keep those products in your shed or on the shelf of your garage. One last note on this, I do not consider myself a gardening expert. I consider myself a biological farmer and gardener.

Now that we've gotten that out of the way, let's start the cleansing of your gardening soul.
Try to imagine gardening without all of that stuff. To let go of what you've been told so far in *A Hundred Years of Deception - Why Gardening Needs to Change*. I hope it's painting a picture worth leaving behind.
If you can see a future where you might not need these things, you might hear a chorus of angels singing because you just opened yourself up to the future of gardening. It's a place where toxins and poisons are relics, and nature and a new form of gardening awaits around the corner to liberate you.

I know that this is scary for many of you as you've trusted the stooges and their websites, shows and blogs for info and gardening techniques and protocols for years. And as far as the liquids, sprays, dust, powders, pellets and crystals, I know your mind is screaming at you, "No, think of the pest infestation next spring!" Or, "My prize roses will die without their 9-12-9 "organic" fertilizer spikes!" Did you know that they were made from feather meal, bone meal and potash? Not organic!

Now, trust me on this, the last piece of your personal, mental garden housecleaning is for you to go online to see when the next poison collection day is for your town or county. You're going to need to know this in the near future for disposing of these toxic substances that you use in your garden.

Isn't it interesting that you'd need to take gardening products to the poison collection sites of your municipality to dispose of them? One last piece as you think about your housecleaning. Did you know that millions of gardeners every year throw their poison into their garbage or recycling bins, and worse their green bins? Yes, millions of pounds of chemical waste from bottles, bags and containers end up in the green yard waste recycling bins every year. How does that sound as an input for your city compost?

As I've said, I am not trying to destroy an industry here, or make you feel bad about a show or a host or an expert you like. I'm trying to change an aspect of a century of gardening that has gone off the cliff on Mr. Toad's Wild Ride. I want you to keep all of the other stuff: the knee pads, netting, trellis', watering cans, potting benches, carts, wheel barrows, aprons, gloves, hats, hoses, irrigation parts, bean poles, tools, tomato cages, rose pruners, loppers, and the other ancillary stuff that feeds the gardening industry and actually help you in the garden.

If you decide to go down the real organic Healthy Gardening path, you will also have to throw out all of the sprayers, misters and cans if they had any of the stuff that you're taking to poison control in them. They will safely dispose of those items for you.

Now, don't you feel better? I do...

# Chapter 13

## A DINOSAUR'S LAST BREATH

I was standing in the center of a huge convention hall when I heard it. There were thousands of customers, buyers, at one of our biggest distributor trade shows of the year. They were all there to get deals on soil, tools, gadgets, gift items, gloves, hats, buckets, sprayers, bird netting, knee pads, outdoor furniture and fertilizers… There was tons of all of that to be had.

In the fall of 2022 as the lawn and garden distribution trade shows had just ended, I was disheartened. There were more fertilizer, pesticide, repellant and herbicide companies and products than I'd ever seen before. Much of this category of products is now labeled natural and organic, and there were still some of the nasty chemical giants like Bayer, the old aspirin and chemical weapons company, on-hand selling their latest and greatest. There was even a faux organic company started by ex-execs of another poison peddler, who'd started their own fake organic line with their retirement dough and investment from friends and family. They were laughing at us. Making a mockery of organic. It was horrific! Disgusting!

There were hundreds of booths with banners describing product benefits on multicolored cardboard end caps filled neatly with spray bottles of pesticides, bags of soil stacked high on pallets, garden art shimmering under the hall lights and thousands of buyers for independent garden centers who had come to stock their shelves. The show announcer would occasionally speak over the hum of the buying and selling, deal making and travel planning to announce that, "So and so from John Doe Garden Center from Two Cows and a Horse, Idaho just won an iPad. Please come and pick it up at the customer service desk, thank you."

This show was a three day happening. One day to set up your booth and get trained on inputting orders on their computer system, one and a half days of selling to the buyers in your booth and a half day to break down your booth and head home. We have built a lot of sales for our companies over the years at these late summer into fall trade shows. That and slinging 40 pounds of compost over my shoulder and driving hundreds of thousands of miles across the country selling a pallet at a time to nurseries, hardware stores, feed and farm supplies and grow shops. Many of those customers were at this trade show. Still many others did not come to the first show after Covid. And many of the smaller mom and pops never come. That's why I put 287,000 miles on the Prius that I built my company with. No sales... no company! In the world of business, sales is king, and here I was standing on the floor of another trade show, selling, taking orders and moving our companies up the food chain.

As I write this I have just returned with my wife from the last big trade show of the year. We did well, our thirteen year old company has become the industry leader in real organic compost and soils. We are also the only farm made and Non-GMO soil company in America. Non-GMO is printed boldly on our bags and it is something that I am very proud of. It was a several year long battle to finally get the organic certifiers to approve the words "Non-GMO" on our bags.

This is interesting to me because as I wrote earlier, the things labeled as organic are also supposed to be Non-GMO. I think the real issue here is that none of the other soil companies test for GMO's or run Genetic ID's like we do, because most of them are slipping in through the organic cracks of organic certification that I discussed in Chapter 6 and Chapter 8. They are using inputs in their products that are labeled organic, but are absolutely not. As you might see this is quite the conundrum for me and for us at our company. We are real organic, farm made and Non-GMO.

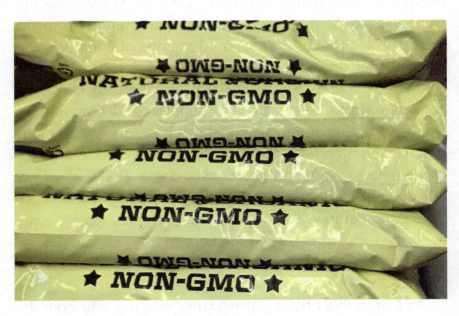

*Organic certifiers approve Non-GMO on our bags*

Everyone else is not! Even the companies who are my friends and allies have products that are, but they also manufacture or label products as organic that are not.

Our own company partnered with a soil engineering firm and demolition contractor to create a second tier line that is certified organic but is not labeled as Non-GMO. It is really good, in fact the second best organic compost and potting soil made in America, and the best topsoil available anywhere. This company is a remediation project of real, actual honest recycling and repurposing, which is the only reason I agreed to do it.

We were asked by a demo contractor friend of mine to test some soil and aged dairy cow manure on a huge site being transitioned from hundred year old dairies to supersites for huge global corporate entities. The topsoil

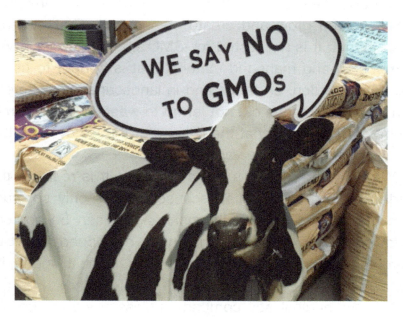

*We Say No to GMO's*

and manure was literally being hauled off and dumped. He believed there had to be a better solution. He didn't think it made any sense to let this natural material go to waste. I went to the site and took bags and bags of soil and aged manure samples and sent them off to the lab. What came back was promising from the toxicology panels, heavy metals analysis and biological assays we ran. The material was clean and would get even better if we could build windrows, bring the biology back to life and heat them up in huge thermophilic windrows. We did and, "Voila" our partnership in that soil company was born.

I shared this with you because that partnership is an example of the future of soil. We can't throw away a century of farming and beneficial biology that was created on the backs and lives of farmers, their families and the animals who gave their service and lives to create healthy food which helped grow and create our country. That material, even though it is not tested for GMO's, is good, clean, well composted and managed material that is perfect to use in the home garden, on farms and in landscapes anywhere. It is a resource that we did not let go to waste. It puts a smile on my face to know that the tail end of the life cycle of that dairy farming was not in vain.

With all that said, it is still a dinosaur. It is roaming this Earth, but has a shelf life because there is only so much clean, safe, and aged dairy manure that can be sourced before all of the old great farmland is developed for tilt-up warehouses and modern housing tracks. Once it's gone, it's gone.

For our original soil company, unless everyone on this planet stops drinking organic dairy products, we will always have a source of real organic and Non-GMO inputs to use in making our compost. We are true recyclers and repurposers who take biologically active living waste and turn it into chocolate brownie colored gold for the soil, your plants, your homegrown food and your garden. One of the very few. It's terrible that, twenty years after organic legislation was outlined by Congress and thirty years after the Organic Food Production Act was passed by Congress, that there are barely any 100% real organic companies selling organic products into the lawn and garden marketplace.

It makes me sad that there aren't fifty companies or a hundred companies like us doing what we do or making products that are 100% real organic. I'm sure that there are some small, local, regional farm companies and soap makers, even bakers or juice companies that make 100% real organic products. I hope so. In truth, I don't know how deeply they test or if the "organic" farms and companies supplying them things to make their organic products test for toxins and GMO's.

In the Big Picture of Big Business, these Big Trade Shows include many brands from Big Ag and Big Chem that still dominate the massive lawn and garden industry. The Big Ag brands are an offshoot of the even larger agriculture industry. These huge chemical companies make garden products because it's extra cash flow. It's also a sneaky way of having you and the government co-sign their poison. Big Distribution gets into the act with fleets of trucks, poly manufacturers who spit out hundreds of millions of bags, bottles and packages, and cardboard companies who blend recycled and non-recycled pulp into boxes that get shipped from point A to point B. Then, it's shipped to point C or D. This is all a huge waste of time, energy and resources. It's a model of business that has become outdated, living past its point of usefulness... It's a dinosaur.

As I said before, I don't want to shut down an industry, I want to awaken the opportunity in front of us to change the path of a giant. A giant that is helping to destroy our environment and foster companies that have no business being in the lawn, garden or agriculture business. I want this industry to be the leader who helps save this planet. I don't agree with Elon Musk that we have to flee Earth. I think we have to save Earth.

All of this input, this download, the methods of gardening and farming I've learned and been perfecting through the use of minimal living inputs over decades, crashed into the dinosaur of lawn and gardening as it exists today on the floor of that last trade show. I heard it again over the buzz and hum of conversation. It was a gasp for air. It grew louder as it gasped again choking for breath. I looked around and realized that I was the only one who'd heard it. It was intended for me to hear, so that I could tell you about it. It was the lawn and garden market taking it's last breath, gasping for air desperately as it fell to the earth... dying!

# Chapter 14

## SMALL THINGS

The old adage that big things come in small packages is true. Some of the greatest gifts, the most important things in life, are small. It's the little things in life that matter. Nothing could be truer.

A little kindness. A little affection. A little attention. A little peace, joy, happiness. These are all things that we could relate to emotionally.

On a hot day a little sip of water is quenching. A little shade when the sun is blistering. A little shelter when it's freezing and cold outside. A little food when we're hungry can change everything, and that my friends is the perfect jumping off point for our transformational tale of David vs. Goliath.

The great biblical story from I Samuel 17 tells of a great story about courage, faith and overcoming the impossible. The story goes like this - The Philistine army was going to war against Israel. The two armies had gathered on hilltops across the valley from each other. A nine foot tall giant Goliath, the greatest warrior of the Philistines, addressed the Philistine army every day for 40 days - mocking Israel and their God. Goliath called the Israelites out to fight, but King Saul and the Israelites were scared, so they did nothing.

A young Israelite named David had gone to the front lines to visit his brothers. He heard Goliath challenge the Israelites and make fun of their God, so David went to King Saul and persuaded him to let him fight Goliath.

Goliath wore armor from head to toe and was armed with a huge sword and spear. He was so intimidating that he put fear into the heart of every man who'd ever seen him. He laughed at the armor-less David as David pronounced that he came in the name of the Lord Almighty, the God of Israel.

David filled his sling with a rock and slung it at the Giant's head. The rock hit the only area that armor wasn't covering Goliath. It sunk into the giant's forehead and he fell to the ground. David picked up Goliath's sword and killed him. Israel had won the war, and the Philistines were under their rule. David's courage and faith saved the nation.

This, better than any story I could think of, is the perfect example of what real organic Healthy Gardening hopes to achieve. The opening chapters of this book have detailed the despicable world created by the giants of the lawn and garden industry - Big Ag, Big Chem, Big Money, Big Trash and Big Gov. They've created and allowed this evil to exist and to thrive. The lawn and garden industry is one that should be clean and healthy and that promotes the best products and practices to help gardeners work and grow in their gardens. Its focus should be on making this Earth more beautiful and abundant.

The days of greenwashing gardeners and of deceiving them with the myth of Fritz Haber and Karl Bosch that have perpetuated into a 121 billion dollar industry in 2022 have come to an end. The 2.1% drop in sales this year is what I believe is the beginning sign of an industry that is starting its decline. It is a dinosaur who doesn't know it yet, but is on its last legs. It is an industry that rakes in, pun intended, $362 per year from every citizen of the U.S. based on the current population of over 332 million people.

That is a ton of dough per person, which is obviously not an accurate picture of who is really buying all of this stuff. It's really you and me, the gardeners who are actually spending a lot more than $362 per year to improve and care for our gardens. I know that my family has.

Notice I use the word has, as in past tense. Why? Because I, my friends and family are the spearhead, the tip of a gardening revolution. We are waking up to face the giant with just small rocks of knowledge and truth. We have changed the way we garden and grow food at home and have quit buying bagged soils, fertilizers, pesticides (natural or not), herbicides (natural or not) and fungicides (natural or not). We have looked at the companies that we buy things from with a critical eye and are vetting them with our wallets now and hitting our Goliath where it hurts him most - the bottom line.

All huge corporations and members of Big anything have boards whose job it is to make sure that whatever board they're sitting on of whatever company they oversee makes as much money as possible. This is the brain of Goliath. His only thought is to sell stuff, make money no matter at what cost or risk to the health and well-being of the people, plants and animals of the Earth. These Goliaths of industry roam the world only to make money, so that profits can be shared and distributed to the shareholders. It's a greed model of more, more and then another heaping helping of

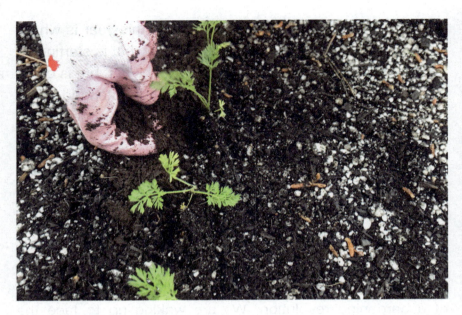
*Composting carrot seedlings using home made compost*

more. It's a sickness that drives many in modern industry. Unfortunately, it almost drives every company, university, church, government and non-profit as well on this planet. It's sad that the world today is under the rule of the greed model and the concept of more.

As I've stated many times in this book, my intention is not to destroy the lawn and garden industry. It is to shine a big spotlight on how messed up it is. How the Haber-Bosch basis of nitrogen fertilization and the fifty year old Cornell University concept of soil re-creation are outdated. It's time for a change. There are still plenty of things that the big distributors can sell you for your garden - soils, fertilizers and pesticides are not one of them.

Hopefully, the distributors will read this book and see it as a breath of fresh air, and one that pushes them to distribute better-made and ecologically-sound products that make the world and our gardens a better place. If nothing else, I hope the distributors realize that soil, fertilizers, pesticides and herbicides are a 1,000 lb. gorilla, actually a 2,000 lb. gorilla, when it comes to a pallet of compost or soil. This is a gorilla that the world can no longer afford because of the high cost of freight and logistics, as well as the environmental implications of cutting down forests for pallets and cardboard and producing millions of pounds of poly for plastic bags and shrink wrap. The world post-Covid is running on all freight, all the time, so much so that trucking companies can't even find enough truckers to fill their fleets of trucks.

## So, How Do We Change Gardening?

Simple! We're going small. We are going to learn how by using small amounts of biology, derived from compost and living soil organisms, that we eliminate a huge piece of the $362 per year slice of Goliath pie. You don't need fertilizers, amendments and bug sprays, or fake organic soils and composts that aren't organic. You need living soil and a garden that is alive with truly natural inputs and ways to grow that are healthy. You also don't need acres of land. You can grow this way on the balcony of an apartment, in a community garden or in a small back yard.

In my follow-up book to *A Hundred Years of Deception — Why Gardening Must Change* I will show you HOW to change gardening. I take you through what I have learned to create a healthy garden and help you transition your garden to a real organic one exactly the way Norma and I grow the gardens on our farm and what we share with our consulting clients. You can get it on Amazon this fall in 2023.

There you will learn to grow lush, productive healthy real organic and Non-GMO gardens through small inoculations (microdoses) of biology, minerals and nutrients for uptake into your plants, your fruits, your veggies, even your prize roses. You will also learn how to successfully grow a healthy garden each season, including how to consciously deal with pests and diseases and how to make Non-GMO, real organic compost and worm castings at home.

There is nothing to fear here except for Goliath — Big CHEM, Big AG, and the Lawn & Garden Manufacturers — who want you to continue believing in the myths and legends of gardening that have held us down for over a hundred years. It's time to take our health and gardens back. The day to change our world with real organic, Non-GMO and chemical-free inputs for a healthy new century and generations beyond is NOW!

Happy and healthy gardening to you from the bottom of my heart...

# Resources

Beytes, Chris. (2018) Behind the Business: Potting Mix—It's in the Bag!. Grower Talks. https://www.growertalks.com/Article/?articleid=23676

Boodley, James W., Sheldrake, Jr., Raymond. (1972). Cornell Peat-Lite Mixes For Commercial Growing. Cornell University Information Bulletin 43. https://ecommons.cornell.edu/bitstream/handle 1813/39084/1972%20Info%20Bulletin%2043.pdf?sequence=2&isAllowed=y

Boodley, James W., Sheldrake, Jr., Raymond. (1982). Cornell Peat-Lite Mixes for Commercial Plant Growing. Cornell University. https://www.vermiculite.org/wp-content/uploads/2014/09/peatlite.pdf

Callie. (2016). Who Invented Potting Mix?. Garden Culture Magazine. http://gardenculturemagazine.com/invented-potting-mix/

Censky, Annalyn. (2020) Pop the cork! Dow ends year up 11%. CNN Money. https://money.cnn.com/2010/12/31/markets/markets_newyork/index.htm

Donley, Nathan, Gunstone, Tari. (2012). Pesticides Are Killing the Organisms That Keep Our Soils Healthy. Scientific American. https://www.scientificamerican.com/article/pesticides-are-killing-the-worlds-soils/

Duca, John. (2013). Subprime Mortgage Crisis 2007–2010. Federal Reserve History. https://www.federalreservehistory.org/essays/subprime-mortgage-crisis

Durfee, Neil. (2018). Holy Crap! A Trip to the World's Largest Guano-Producing Islands. Audobon. https://www.audubon.org/news/holy-crap-trip-worlds-largest-guano-producing-islands

Formuzis, Alex. (2022). Environmental Working Group. Internal papers show Syngenta hid risks of widely used pesticide from public, regulators for decades. https://www.ewg.org/news-insights/news-release/2022/11/internal-papers-show-syngenta-hid-risks-widely-used-pesticide

Grubinger, Vern. (2012). POTTING MIXES FOR ORGANIC GROWERS. University of Vermont Extension. https://www.uvm.edu/vtvegandberry/factsheets/pottingmix.html

Gwartney, James D., Connors, Joseph. (2009). National Council for the Social Studies.https://www.uwp.edu/learn/departments/economics/upload/gwartney-summary-of-financial-crisis.pdf

Halley, Jim. (2023). After Dropping Nearly 70%, Is It Time to Buy Scotts Miracle-Gro Stock Yet? The Motley Fool. https://www.fool.com/investing/2023/01/05/after-dropping-nearly-70-is-it-time-to-buy-scotts/

Harford, Tim. (2017). How fertiliser helped feed the world. BBC News.
https://www.bbc.com/news/business-38305504

Klaslow, Lee. (2022). Five charts on US trucking: 2023 outlook. Bloomberg. https://www.bloomberg.com/professional/blog/five-charts-on-us-trucking-2023-outlook/

Lingenfelter, Dwight, William, S. Curran. (2021). Guidelines for Weed Management in Roundup® Ready Alfalfa. Penn State Extension. https://extension.psu.edu/guidelines-for-weed-management-in-roundup-ready-alfalfa/

Long, Mindy. (2022) Shippers Remain in Control of Rates, but 2023 Could Bring Balance. Transport Topics. https://www.ttnews.com/articles/shippers-remain-control-rates-2023-could-bring-balance

Mineral Products Industry. (1995). Perlite Processing. https://www3.epa.gov/ttnchie1/ap42/ch11/final/c11s30.pdf

Newman, Julie. Core facts about coir. Nursery Magazine. https://www.nurserymag.com/article/core-facts-about-coir/

Nigro, Dana. (2014). Remembering a Guru of Green: Biodynamic Consultant Alan York. https://www.winespectator.com/articles/remembering-a-guru-of-green-biodynamic-consultant-alan-york-49613

Pokorny, Kym. (2022). Harvesting pea moss contributes to climate change, Oregon State scientist says. https://today.oregonstate.edu/news/harvesting-peat-moss-contributes-climate-change

Royal Horticutural Society. Peat-free compost choices. https://www.rhs.org.uk/soil-composts-mulches/peat-free

Souraya, Sakoui, Derdak, Reda, Boutaina, Addoum, Serrano-Delgado, Aurelio, Soukri, Abdelaziz, Bouchra, El Khalfi. (2020). The Life Hidden Inside Caves: Ecological and Economic Importance of Bat Guano. Hindawi. https://www.hindawi.com/journals/ijecol/2020/9872532/

Statista. (2023). Lawn & Garden - United States. https://www.statista.com/outlook/cmo/diy-hardware-store/lawn-garden/united-states

Supply Chain Management Review. (2022). Supply chain issues not over yet
A survey by SAP SE shows that global unrest and costs will continue as major problems. https://www.scmr.com/article/supply_chain_issues_not_over_yet

Trafton, Anne. (2020). Technique could enable cheaper fertilizer production.. MIT News. https://news.mit.edu/2020/cheaper-fertilizer-production-0504

Trail, Jesse Vernon. (2013). The truth about peat moss. Ecologist. https://theecologist.org/2013/jan/25/truth-about-peat-moss

Tyson, Jim. (2022). Recession likely in 2023, Fitch says. CFO Dive. https://www.cfodive.com/news/recession-likely-2023-fitch-says/631647/

U.S. Food & Drug Administration. (2022). GMO Crops, Animal Food, and Beyond. https://www.fda.gov/food/agricultural-biotechnology/gmo-crops-animal-food-and-beyond

Whitney, Todd. (2021). Pasture and Forage Minute: Alfalfa Weeds and Thinning Stands. University of Nebraska-Lincoln. Cropwatch. https://cropwatch.unl.edu/2021/pasture-and-forage-alfalfa-weeds-and-thinning-stands

Wood, Laura. (2022). Global Lawn and Garden Consumables Market (2022 to 2027) - Industry Trends, Share, Size, Growth, Opportunity and Forecasts - ResearchAndMarkets.com https://www.businesswire.com/news/home/20220408005362/en/Global-Lawn-and-Garden-Consumables-Market-2022-to-2027---Industry-Trends-Share-Size-Growth-Opportunity-and-Forecasts---ResearchAndMarkets.com

Wyenandt, Andy, Nitzsche, Peter. (2020). Rutgers. https://njaes.rutgers.edu/fs547/

Yiu, Enoch, Bray, Chad. (2021) South China Morning Post. Syngenta, Swiss agrochemicals giant owned by ChemChina, kick-starts process to list Shanghai's Star Market. https://www.scmp.com/business/banking-finance/article/3138222/chemchina-owned-250-year-old-swiss-agrichemicals-giant

# About the Author

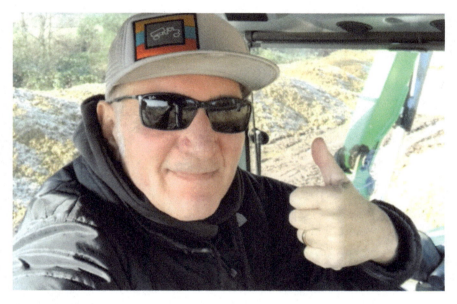

Randy Ritchie is a member of the Writer's Guild of America and was a screenwriter and landscaper before he created the first eco-landscape company in Los Angeles. His search for real, living, healthy organic compost led him to create Malibu Compost. He has taught real organic gardening to tens of thousands of gardeners across America and at national garden shows and now teaches online to reach more people. Ritchie offers consulting services to home gardeners, estate horticulturists, hotel managers, farmers, landscapers, urban farmers and homesteaders. He is the host of the weekly podcast, The Healthy Garden.

Made in the USA
Las Vegas, NV
18 November 2024

12083596R00066